What people are saying about …

Her Choice to Heal

"For women who suffer from the emotional aftermath of abortion, *Her Choice to Heal* is a wellspring of healing waters. This is not a book to be read, but a book to be experienced. With deep empathy, Sydna Massé offers hope to those women who suffer from the emotional pain following an abortion. She points the way to healing through Christ."

Gary D. Chapman, author of *The Five love Languages* and *Love as a Way of Life*

"In your neighborhood, your office, or in the church pew next to you, there are women who are silently suffering from the pain of a choice they made to end the life of an unborn child. It may have been years ago or just a few days ago. You may know the pain yourself. This is a book that can begin the process of healing the ache in your soul."

Bob Lepine, cohost of FamilyLife Today

"The author cut right to the core of the personal turmoil a woman experiences after an abortion. Hope is given in a simple, step-by-step approach that assures women everywhere that they can find healing from these spiritual and emotional wounds."

Beverly LaHaye, chair of Concerned Women for America

"God is using Sydna Massé's wou this church who are suffering fror *to Heal* is an astonishing work of practical advice."

Gary Thomas, author of *Sacred Marriage*

"*Her Choice to Heal* gives life-changing insight into the struggles of post-abortive women. This book will also allow men to better understand and more effectively help their wives with some of the resulting battles abortion causes. This brief book is extremely sensitive, practical, and comprehensive. But more than that, it is a story of God's love and forgiveness for all of us who have made poor choices. Sydna's love and passion is revealed by her vulnerability in sharing her personal journey to healing."

Dr. Clarence Shuler, president/CEO of
Building Lasting Relationships, Inc.

"*Her Choice to Heal* is a rare tool in helping women who are struggling with the pain that often follows an abortion decision. Through Meier Clinics, we are increasingly coming into contact with post-abortive men and women who need direct ministry in grieving these children and coming to a point of peace through God's redemptive love. This book is a great tool to help these clients understand the system we employ in processing this pain and move forward in embracing the healing that God provides."

Paul Meier, MD, founder of Meier Clinics

"Acknowledging the effect abortion has had on your life and seeking help can be really difficult, particularly if you are a Christian. Guilt can lock women and men into silence and despair. However, at CareConfidential we have seen many women work through painful emotions and experience God's love and forgiveness and so able to face their future with hope and peace. With two hundred thousand abortions every year in the United Kingdom, many more need to hear this message. From her own experience of abortion, pain, and healing, Sydna Massé offers hope to many."

Joanna Thompson, executive director of CareConfidential, UK

"The word *abortion* brings judgment, shame, heartache, and defensiveness to the surface. The war regarding abortion is intense and dark and is seldom addressed with the clarity, compassion, and conviction of God's mercy as found in this excellent book. Sydna Massé has offered those who have experienced abortion firsthand and those who love them a wise and kind path for healing. She is honest, hopeful, and passionately convinced that the love of God is stronger than death, and transformation surer than shame. I am profoundly grateful for this labor of love."

Dan B. Allender, PhD, president and professor of
Counseling Psychology, Mars Hill Graduate School and
author of *The Wounded Heart* and *The Healing Path*

"Even though I've never had an abortion, this book has helped me. A must read for post-abortive women."

Norma McCorvey, (Roe of Roe v. Wade) author of *Won By Love*

"I first read *Her Choice to Heal* while on a plane trip ten years ago. As a post-abortive woman, it didn't take too long for tears to come as I read the testimony of Sydna Massé. There isn't a better resource for women who are beginning to look at this pain in their lives. In my recent work to end abortion in South Dakota, as well as my leadership at the National Abstinence Clearinghouse and the Alpha Center for Women in Sioux Falls, South Dakota, I know that post-abortion healing is a key element in stopping abortion from devastating our society. Without hearing our testimonies of pain, the world will continue to believe that abortion is a good choice."

Leslee Unruh, president and founder of the National
Abstinence Clearinghouse, abstinence.net

"A valuable contribution to tearing down the stone wall that too many women have built in order to hide the truth and the shame."

Cal Thomas, syndicated columnist

"For those of you who have struggled with the guilt and shame of abortion, this book offers hope and healing. God's blessing to Sydna for her courage to speak to the broken-hearted."

Kathy Troccoli, recording artist

"*Her Choice to Heal* is the classic companion for the post-abortion journey, and so much more. For years, it's been the ultimate source of deeply personal insights, practical help, and ultimate hope for hurting women and those who love them. And now, after all these years of leading the way, I'm can't wait to see this revised and updated edition impact a whole new generation!"

Mark Andrew Olsen, author of *Hadassah,*
The Road Home, and *The Watchers*

"Through the loss of my husband, Keith Green, and two of our young children in a plane crash, I am intimately aware of God's tender mercy and care for those who grieve. A few years after Keith's death I started Americans Against Abortion as the pro-life arm of Last Day's Ministries. How I wish Sydna's book had been available back then as we took part in pioneering the pro-life movement across the nation. In *Her Choice to Heal,* Sydna shares the clear hope that God can forgive and redeem the pain suffered after an abortion. If you or someone you know has experienced this tragedy, I highly recommend this book."

Melody Green, president of Last Days Ministries and author of
No Compromise: The Life Story of Keith Green (Legacy Edition)

her choice to heal

.her
choice
to heal

Finding
Spiritual and
Emotional Peace
After Abortion

Sydna Massé

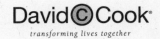

David C Cook®
transforming lives together

HER CHOICE TO HEAL
Published by David C. Cook
4050 Lee Vance View
Colorado Springs, CO 80918 U.S.A.

David C. Cook Distribution Canada
55 Woodslee Avenue, Paris, Ontario, Canada N3L 3E5

David C. Cook U.K., Kingsway Communications
Eastbourne, East Sussex BN23 6NT, England

David C. Cook and the graphic circle C logo
are registered trademarks of Cook Communications Ministries.

The Web site addresses recommended throughout this book are offered as a
resource to you. These Web sites are not intended in any way to be or imply an
endorsement on the part of David C. Cook, nor do we vouch for their content.

Some of the names in this book have been changed to protect the privacy of the individuals.

All Scripture quotations, unless otherwise noted, are taken from the *Holy Bible, New
International Version*®. *NIV*®. Copyright © 1973, 1978, 1984 by International Bible
Study. Used by permission of Zondervan. All rights reserved. Scripture quotations
marked NKJV taken from the New King James Version. Copyright © 1982 by Thomas
Nelson, Inc. Used by permission. All rights reserved; TLB taken from *The Living Bible*,
© 1971, Tyndale House Publishers, Wheaton, IL 60189. Used by permission.

LCCN 2008938712
ISBN 978-1-4347-6872-8

© 2009 Sydna Massé

First edition published by Chariot Victor Publishing in 1998 ©
Sydna Massé and Joan Phillips. ISBN 1-56476-734-5.

The Team: Terry Behimer, Melanie Larson, Amy Kiechlin, Jaci Schneider, and Karen Athen
Cover Design: ThinkPen Design, Greg Jackson
Cover Illustration: istockphoto

Printed in the United States of America
Second Edition 2009

5 6 7 8 9 10 11 12 13 14

110409

If you know someone who's had an abortion ...

Do you have a friend or relative who has had an abortion? Maybe you were involved in her decision from the outset ... maybe you were in the waiting room during the procedure ... maybe she confided in you long after the fact. However you found out, you picked up this book because you care, because you've seen her sadness and wondered how to help.

Your best gift to her will be your love and prayers. She may or may not be ready to work through her pain. But perhaps this book can be a resource—something she can tuck in a drawer and pull out some rainy day when the issue has become too hard to avoid. When that day comes, be ready with a list of "positive-life" groups—those who do not express judgment toward individuals who have made this choice but are warm and compassionate—such as pregnancy care centers, post-abortion ministries, and other resources in your community. These can usually be found in the "abortion alternatives" section of your yellow pages or online at RamahInternational.org. But most of all, be ready with your unconditional support. God bless you in your desire to help.

If you have had an abortion ...

Perhaps you are thinking, *Okay, so I had an abortion. But that's in my past. Do I really need to be healed?*

Some women seemingly never need to work through any kind of healing process. But for many of us, the memory of abortion lies like a hidden infection within, weakening and impairing us in ways we may have never realized were related. Is that true for you? See if you recognize yourself in some of the following questions. (A more complete list appears on pages 50–55.)

- Do you avoid the subject of abortion, or do you feel guilt, anger, or sorrow when remembering or discussing your own abortion?
- Do you tend to think of your life in terms of "before" and "after" the abortion?
- Do you have lingering feelings of resentment or anger toward people involved in your abortion, such as the baby's father, your friends, or your parents?
- Have you found yourself either avoiding relationships or becoming overly dependent in them since the abortion? Are you overly protective of any children you have now?
- Have you begun or increased use of drugs or alcohol since the abortion, or do you have an eating disorder?
- Have you felt a vague sort of emptiness, a deep sense of loss, or had prolonged periods of depression?
- Do you sometimes have nightmares or flashbacks relating to the abortion?
- Are you concerned about your ability to get pregnant in the future?

If so, it is likely you are experiencing post-abortion syndrome. God's relief and healing can be found for you in the pages of this book. I invite you to read on and find the peace you had forgotten existed.

If you are considering abortion …

Abortion is presented to women as a safe and legal option. Rarely are individuals offered information about the very real consequences of this choice.

Regardless of your reasons for considering abortion, please understand that there is a strong possibility that you may regret this decision at a psychological, spiritual, emotional, or even physical level. Abortion results in pregnancy loss, which can eventually result in emotions such as grief, guilt, and shame. Most psychological associations don't recognize abortion pain as a pregnancy loss issue. Others diminish the risks by saying that abortion is easier and safer than childbirth. Post-abortive women are too afraid of society's judgment to take a stand and demand new research efforts that will outline that their pain does exist and is related to their abortion decision. After speaking to thousands of individuals over the years, in all types of situations, it has been obvious that abortion hurts most hearts in many unrecognized ways at some point in their lives. I urge you to read further and learn more about all aspects of abortion pain before you make a choice you may regret for the rest of your life.

Contact your local pregnancy care center for support, information, and assistance. These positive-life groups are caring, confidential, complimentary, and nonjudgmental. Many of these centers are staffed by individuals who have also experienced an unplanned pregnancy. These organizations can usually be found in the "abortion alternatives" section of your yellow pages or online at RamahInternational.org.

How to read this book ...

The peace you search for will come, but it may not come quickly or all at once. Read this book slowly. You may read a chapter, and then spend days or weeks processing what you have read. Consider employing different ways of working through the information. Writing is a form of self-expression, self-examination, and self-therapy.

Many times it is difficult to know what you are thinking and feeling until you put it in writing. You can visit RamahInternational.org for chapter-by-chapter ideas and insights that can help you get started. It might also help to keep a journal of your ideas, thoughts, and prayers during this time. Others express their emotions through artwork, poetry, gardening, or music. Just remember, there are no boundaries, no rights or wrongs about how or what to write. Use whatever form of expression helps you most.

Others of you may need to find a person to confide in, someone who can be trusted with your deepest fears and secrets. A friend who has stood by you in the past, perhaps, or a professional counselor can help in the process. For help in finding someone to talk to, call the pregnancy care center in your town. (See "abortion alternatives" section in the yellow pages directory or visit RamahInternational.org.)

This book is lovingly dedicated to Jesse Hawthorne Massé, whose death has been redeemed many times through the wonderful love, grace, and mercy of Jesus Christ.

Contents

Acknowledgments

My deepest thanks goes to my family, whose personal encouragement has enabled this book to be written. To the most important people in my life: my husband, Thomas, who has always stood quietly by my side in supporting every element of outreach, providing godly counsel, spiritual leadership, and magnificent love and patience; my three sons, Bruce, Michael, and Daniel, who continue to provide their permission and blessing on the work God has called me to do, teaching me new things every day and filling my heart with love; my mother, Mary McLachlin, and my adopted father, Mac—Bruce Robert McLachlin—who recently passed into God's heavenly care where they are finally enjoying their first grandson.

Finally, I am grateful to each person who has assisted us in this project and for the prayers of the faithful that have inspired this work.

I am also most appreciative to the dedicated board of directors of Ramah International, who have supported me over the years, as well as the endorsers of this book, who believe in post-abortion pain as a real issue in our society today.

My thanks also go to Dr. Clarence Shuler, who has been my friend for so many years, providing amazing insight and wisdom into this field, particularly with addressing men's post-abortion pain.

I'm grateful to Tammy Hoelting, Karen Fifer, Vikki Parker, Nona Hoard Stafford, Nancy Knowlton, and Joann Tallman for their love, friendship, and godly support over these many years.

There are countless others to thank as well—especially those of you who have traipsed around the world with me to offer the hope of God's healing. You know who you are!

To Dr. Vincent Rue and Dr. David Reardon, for sharing years of research and analysis. To Dr. Paul and Teri Reisser, who initially outlined post-abortion syndrome as a form of post-traumatic stress disorder. To Linda Cochrane, who authored the study that God used to help me, and so many others, find His healing love. I am humbled by the generosity of these people. Without their dedication and compassion for the post-abortive individual, the truth might never be known of the devastating effects abortion has on the human race.

My gratitude goes out to amazing pregnancy care centers and post-abortion programs all over the world that continue to show abortion-vulnerable and post-abortive women the unconditional love of Christ. Without the compassion, understanding, and support of the trained counselors at a local pregnancy care centers, I may not have had the courage to face the truth and found God's healing and peace. May God greatly bless and multiply your efforts.

I would like to thank Dr. James C. Dobson of Focus on the Family. You were one of the first Christian leaders to publicly recognize the pain a woman can feel after an abortion. Because of your faithfulness in this area, many of us are now living fruitful lives, becoming better wives, daughters, sisters, aunts, and mothers.

To Rev. H. B. London Jr., thank you, dear friend. You allowed me to benefit from your wonderful pastoral leadership when I first began my work with pregnancy care centers. Thank you for believing in me and offering compassion to the millions of women who still sit in silent prisons of pain after an abortion loss.

To the staff at David C. Cook—initially Lee Hough and now

Melanie Larson—who gave godly insight and wisdom, along with many heartfelt prayers—I couldn't have done this without you!

In closing, I would like to thank you, the reader of this book, for caring enough to look at this issue either in your own heart or for those who are around you. You have begun a journey that God will lead specifically and use you to minister His love to others!

Foreword

She walked into my office. I could tell she was nervous. When I heard her story I could tell why. She was post-abortive, she had a new boyfriend and was afraid to tell him her story. She loved the church, but felt people would shun her when they found out about her past. Besides that it was almost the birthday time for her aborted child and she was feeling very guilty ... and sad.

You might think this story unique, but when you serve the church and walk in the village for very long, you soon learn that those with stories like the one above are everywhere. I have also learned that there are times when you can help these desperate people, but unfortunately many times you cannot. I have struggled over the reasons why so many do not let the church and others help.

One of the thoughts that seems most logical is they just do not want to hurt anymore. The wound is still fresh. The memories too vivid. I have heard them ask over and over, "Who can I trust?" "Will I be betrayed?" "Can I ever feel like a whole person again?" "Why are people so judgmental?" You might understand if they were referring to the "world," but that is not the case. Most of the time they are making reference to the church.

I think, as a pastor, I was there for a while. The thought of ending the life of God's creation was abhorrent to me. The whole idea was unimaginable. From the pulpit I would make my case for life, and do it in such a way that innocently, I was not only offending many, but making life more difficult for those who were dealing with the guilt and loss that accompanies abortion. Until one day another young lady helped me to see the error of my preaching. From that time until now my distaste for abortion has not changed, but my love and consideration for those who have experienced this devastating procedure has grown.

Some in spiritual leadership must feel that the stronger and more condemning their rhetoric against abortion is, the more people will be influenced to choose morality and chastity. I pray that be so, but for most who hear the bombastic sermons, it only causes more pain and a tendency to withdraw even further into one's private hell. I apologize for those who inflict pain rather than healing. Pastor, please be gentle, loving, and forgiving. Offer hope, not despair—even as Jesus our Great Shepherd would do.

As I read the pages of *Her Choice to Heal*, I think back to the early days of Sydna's passion to help those who had been wounded even as she had. I think back to those countless hours we sat together discussing how she could establish a vehicle for God to use in reaching the post-abortive. And then one day, like a little bird finding its wings, she just took off and her work with Ramah International began.

So much of what Sydna does is a step of faith. What keeps her going I'm not sure, but I imagine it to be the support she receives from her family, the anointing God has placed upon her, and the fruit of her labor. She has seen the results of her investment—changed lives, healed emotions, and freedom to love again restored to countless numbers.

I would go so far as to say when you read the wisdom with which Sydna writes, and the emotion that flows from her heart for those like her who have felt the sting of moral failure and wondered if life would ever be normal again … it will change you and sensitize your understanding forevermore.

"Then neither do I condemn you," Jesus declared. "Go now and leave your life of sin" (John 8:11).

Rev. H. B. London Jr.
Vice President, Church & Clergy
Focus on the Family

Prologue

Since the January 22, 1973, *Roe v. Wade* Supreme Court decision, which legalized abortion in the United States, there have been an average of 1.2 million abortions every year—and for every one of those abortions, a mother found herself faced with a painful decision and the physical and emotional stress of the procedure itself. At least half of American women will experience an unintended pregnancy by age forty-five, and, at current rates, about one-third will have had an abortion. Of these post-abortive women, 47 percent of them have had at least one previous abortion.[1]

At first many women feel relief. They no longer are faced with the problem of an unplanned or unwanted pregnancy. Some will go through another unplanned pregnancy, perhaps aborting again and again and again. For months or even years, the only apparent truth is that the woman made the right decision for that time in her life.

But underlying those feelings of relief are often other feelings that are quite unexplained. Feelings of loss, guilt, and confusion seem to persist for no apparent reason. Life seems to be a roller coaster of emotion, with extreme highs and lows. Many women turn to substance abuse to ease or hide this inexplicable pain that persistently nags at their souls.

Other women avoid the pain by undergoing an emotional desensitization, or "numbing." Working hard to keep their feelings in check, they experience neither highs nor lows. For some women this creates a callousness, a lack of sensitivity, which hampers their ability to form and maintain close interpersonal relationships.

Although abortion is legally and socially acceptable in most countries, society still attaches a stigma to it. Most women never talk about their abortions and try not to think about them. Abortion is usually considered best forgotten by all involved. Fearful of being exposed, judged, condemned, and/or rejected, a woman commonly finds herself withdrawing deeper within herself, telling herself that as long as no one finds out, she can go on with life as if nothing ever happened.

But something did happen. Her body was invaded. A child was taken from the sanctuary of her womb, a place that is supposed to be the ultimate in safety and security. And, as much as she wants to believe that she has had a mere lump of tissue removed in a simple medical procedure, some deep part of her knows that is not the truth. Although well-meaning people assured her that the ordeal would soon be behind her, for most women that is not the case. Most will suffer deeply and silently, in broad-spread ways. The symptoms that they have are known as post-abortion syndrome (PAS), which is based on the well-recognized psychological disorder post-traumatic stress disorder (PTSD).

Research by David Reardon of the Elliott Institute has shown that, regardless of age, family size, race, marital status, or number of abortions, of those surveyed,

- 61 percent experience flashbacks
- 54 percent have anniversary reactions
- 33 percent feel suicidal
- 78 percent have feelings of diminished control of their lives
- 52 percent experience difficulty developing and maintaining relationships
- 49 percent begin or increase drug use[2]

Ironically, though women seek out abortion as a solution to stressful circumstances, abortion itself can become a contributor to long-lasting stress of a different kind.

As someone who has experienced firsthand the lasting effects of abortion, I know that post-abortion syndrome does, indeed, exist, but that it can be overcome. To the woman who is struggling, I would like to extend to you my compassion—as well as a supporting arm to guide you along the way to healing through the pages of this book.

For those of you who have experienced abortion multiple times, the pain may have intensified with each choice. Your healing process can be different in that you may need to address each lost child on an individual basis. Throughout this book, when I say "child" I will be referring to each one of your aborted children, because each loss is unique, special, and significant in the eyes of the Lord. You are in my prayers as you begin your journey toward peace.

Chapter 1

My Abortion Story

*Then I heard a loud voice saying in heaven, "Now
salvation, and strength, and the kingdom of our God,
and the power of His Christ have come, for the accuser
of our brethren, who accused them before our God day
and night, has been cast down. And they overcame
him by the blood of the Lamb and by the word of
their testimony, and they did not love their lives to the
death. Therefore rejoice, O heavens, and you who dwell
in them! Woe to the inhabitants of the earth and the
sea! For the devil has come down to you, having great
wrath, because he knows that he has a short time."*
—Revelation 12:10–12 NKJV

No one experiences an abortion in a bubble. Most of us have a
background of trauma that often leads to sexual activity outside of

marriage and eventually an unwanted pregnancy. This unplanned pregnancy can occur within a marriage as well. In understanding this pain, you must begin to look at your life before and after the abortion. Choices others made for you or that you made yourself could have made you vulnerable to an abortion decision. Most of us did not make this choice in a "murderous" mind-set, but in a fearful state, not necessarily considering other choices.

God sees our lives as part of this huge incredible tapestry that is all woven together, from generation to generation. Our human eyes, however, often see only the messy backside of our own tiny piece of that tapestry, with its intermittent and jumbled threads. We concentrate on our pain and can't see how the Lord could take our tragedies and turn them for His good. You'll hear me say this several times, because I want you to remember it: God never wastes our pain and He will make good use of every past experience in your future life.

Post-Abortive Women Among Us

Since entering the field of unplanned pregnancy and post-abortion outreach in 1991, I have had the great blessing of working with multitudes of post-abortive individuals at all stages of healing. We are everywhere—in churches, shopping centers, grocery stores, daycare centers, high schools, pregnancy centers. We encompass all spectrums of the educational system, from high school dropouts to PhD holders. We often work well below our level of capacity or at the top levels of corporations, governments, and institutions.

Statistics from abortion providers say that if you look into any American audience, nearly one third of the women you see could have experienced an abortion.[1]

Abortion is the most common form of surgical procedure in the United States, yet also the one that is rarely discussed in any setting. For most of us, abortion is a secret we dare not share. We think that if people—even loved ones—knew about our abortion decision, they would not like us, love us, or associate with us. In the unhealed heart of many post-abortive women, we have committed a sin that is so horrendous, we believe it to be unforgivable. This sin stamps a scarlet letter A on our foreheads and souls.

Society is not going to punish us. We punish ourselves with self-destructive behaviors: drugs, alcohol, eating disorders, sexual dysfunctions, suicide attempts or completions, abusive relationships—often never associating this pain and behavior with our abortion decision. That memory is buried so deeply and covered with other dysfunctional activities in an attempt to distance our minds from the seemingly haunting presence of our lost children.

Somewhere along this road, though, something snaps, and we can no longer bear the burden of these memories. Perhaps the break is triggered on the anniversary of the *Roe v. Wade* decision, when abortion is often featured in media channels. Or it could be a Mother's Day celebration. Getting pregnant and giving birth is an overwhelming reminder. Or perhaps it is in a second, third, fourth unplanned pregnancy, where abortion is repeated. Hearing a song from that period or a fragrance can remind us of the moment when we lost so much. Yearly anniversary dates, such as the date of the abortion or the due date of the child, can also initiate this depression.

When these triggers of pain occur, some confess—perhaps quietly, discreetly, tentatively, or even angrily to a friend, loved one, or family member. The pain is obvious, and the relief in finally stepping out to recognize our lost children is the first step in the healing process.

But others dare not confess and further withdraw into themselves, trusting no one. They have overheard conversations portraying painful condemnations, such as "I don't know how anyone could ever choose abortion. They must be horrible people." Even in approaching the abortion clinic, some were branded and taunted by certain types of abortion opponents. Those voices propelled us into the apparently safe arms of those who assisted us in this choice we would come to regret so deeply.

In this book you will read my story of healing, wholeness, and the joy in Christ that came through mourning my child lost through abortion. You may recognize your own pain in these words. My prayer is that the Lord will use my typical story to comfort you, to help you realize that you are not alone in the emotions you experience, that you are not going crazy, and that you can be forgiven.

My Story

When I was a child, my father was a well-respected minister at a conservative, Bible-believing church. I was proud of him, especially when people would flock down the aisle after his sermons to find a new life in Christ.

I remember when a congregation member patted my head and said, "Someday you are going to be quite the wild young girl, Sydna." I was shocked at his conclusion and spoke in my own defense, relaying that I loved the Lord and would never be that way. He simply laughed and said, "Wait and see. All preachers' kids are wild. Your day will come."

My parents' marriage was never stable or obviously loving, but I had no idea that there was any sort of problem. My father was away conducting important church business—I never dreamed he was involved in extramarital affairs, including one with my best friend's mother. My mother realized the possibility but determined to ignore these "potential" infidelities for the sake of his ministry.

In 1972, I was eleven, and my father began to counsel a woman who began to develop a strong hold on him. When a bond between them grew obvious, my mother couldn't ignore the situation any more. She gave him an ultimatum: her or the other woman—my father chose the other woman. When my mother threatened divorce, which would have ended his career, my father had her quickly committed to a mental health facility due to a "nervous breakdown."

For that entire summer, I rarely saw my mother and lived with a friend because my father's attention to the new woman left him no time to care for me. My older brother had been sent away on a mission trip. The church took notice of my father's continuous absence from his pastoral duties, and he was forced to resign. Once free of the mental institution, my mother filed for divorce. My brother decided to live with our father, so my mother lost both her husband and son during that period—I lost a father and a brother.

Around this time, my best friend's mother came to help us move into our new home. I didn't yet know about her infidelity with my father.

This woman took me aside and said, "I need to ask for your forgiveness, Sydna." No adult was ever so serious with me, so I listened attentively. She went on to say, "I was sexually involved with your father and I need to confess that to you and ask for your forgiveness. Will you forgive me?"

Shock and embarrassment set into my heart immediately as I visually pictured them locked in a passionate embrace. All I could offer was a nod, which she interpreted as forgiveness. She hugged me and left me alone. I was changed in that moment and struggled to rid my mind of the horrendous thoughts of them together. Unsure whether my mother knew this truth about her friend and my father, I never mentioned the confession to her. This woman's burden of sin had just been transferred to my eleven-year-old shoulders.

Finally, the lie that had been my father's ministry life exploded into my world, tearing it to shreds. As understanding dawned with me, a scandal exploded when my father's sexual escapades became known in the community. My mother pretended not to be bothered by the scandal, often saying, "We'll show them all, Sydna. They'll know I'm a good mother because you are going to turn out wonderful." I was incredibly broken, but became my mother's emotional support, vowing to be perfect so that I would never hurt her.

My father never had any real sort of presence in my life after that. Over the years, he would see me only about once a month. I hated those visits because they often left me feeling empty and unloved, ugly and undesirable. Even if he had been more attentive, the damage was complete between us.

A few years later my mother married her boss, Bruce, who did not embrace her belief in Jesus. This stepfather, who would later legally adopt me, provided financial stability to our broken home. Bruce, whom we called "Mac," provided some magnificent strength to my mother's life and adored me. While he didn't initially share our faith, he would go to church each Sunday in an attempt to understand our spiritual perspective. Mac would help me with homework and defend me in all arguments. He never tried to replace my dad but just tried to be a "fatherly" friend. Nevertheless, as I approached the later stages of adolescence, the wildness predicted years before began....

End of Innocence

In a turn of irony, I lost my virginity while attending a conservative abstinence seminar. Clearly, I wasn't listening to any of the teachings but instead focusing on the boy who held my heart—I thought I was in love. I had just graduated high school and wanted my first time to be with someone special.

We had pushed all the limits of sexual activity for months until we finally determined to cross the line. After that one encounter, I endured my first real pregnancy scare. When my period finally arrived, the relationship ended.

During my second semester of college at a private Christian university, I found myself missing my ex-boyfriend, and I had yet to make any real friends among the girls in my dorm. I was miserable at school and desperately lonely. So when Alan began to pursue a relationship with me, he seemed like my knight in shining armor. He was the son of a minister as well and could understand my emotions as a preacher's kid. Alan was truly wild, smoking pot and drinking heavily.

I knew his attraction to me was primarily superficial. But then again, I was attracted to him for the escape he provided from my loneliness. His friends were very popular, and they became my friends as well. There was only one catch to the relationship—sex. Since I wasn't a virgin anyway, it didn't seem to be too high a price to pay to keep Alan around, despite the fact that I never enjoyed our physical encounters. Still, using birth control would have made the whole thing seem too deliberate … and that summer, I found myself pregnant.

Alan was adamant that abortion was our only choice. Knowing my mother simply couldn't endure the agony of another public scandal, I had to agree with him. I wouldn't put her through that pain, I reasoned. Abortion was best for everyone.

Alan waited in the car when I went for the pregnancy test at the local family planning clinic. My whole world turned upside down when the woman confirmed that I was pregnant. Through tears, I told her that as a "good Christian girl" I had no other choice but abortion, and she helped me schedule an appointment at a clinic close to my school. I didn't know anything about abortion except that many of my girlfriends had made the choice. They came back seemingly fine, mostly relieved, and not obviously traumatized.

Deep inside, though, I was beginning to fall in love with my unborn baby, and as I left the office, I dared to hope Alan might support me in this pregnancy. When he saw my tear-stained face and realized I was indeed pregnant, he read my mind and quietly said, "If you are thinking of continuing this pregnancy, Sydna, let me lay out the situation for you. I will tell everyone it's not mine, and I will not allow my parents to help you. Your mother will have a nervous breakdown. The school doesn't allow pregnant unwed students, so you'll be kicked out. You'll be on your own! It doesn't look like you have much choice. Plus, I was on acid the night it was conceived, so it would probably come out handicapped anyway."

Once again, I felt hopelessly alone and backed into a corner. I also thought that if the father was so willing to reject his child, the baby would be better off not being brought into the world. I knew the pain of my own father's abandonment and didn't want that for any of my children. Never did I consider how much I would miss that child for the rest of my life.

The Abortion

I began to distance myself from any maternal feelings I might have toward my unborn child. Since I was only four weeks along, I was informed that I would have to wait three weeks to ensure that the procedure was "successful." As I waited, I forced myself to view this child as the enemy that would end my mother's sanity and my security. I also hoped that perhaps I would have a future with Alan; that this abortion would be something that might bring us closer together in future months—I didn't know that the majority of couples who choose abortion break up eventually. Around this time, I began to join him in smoking pot and drinking. I even tried LSD right before my abortion. These actions cemented the abortion decision because I knew the fetus could be harmed by my drug use—but since this child wasn't going to be born, my behavior didn't seem to matter.

I remember trying to get my mother's attention in those weeks, hoping she would ask me if something was wrong. My heart wanted to share the truth and have this child become part of our lives. Yet I was afraid she would withdraw her support for my education, send me away to avoid additional scandal, and force me to place my baby for adoption, which seemed far more brutal than abortion. Adoption had always horrified me. If I had the strength to parent, certainly I would never give my child away. Never once did I realize that adoption would mean my child could *live*. All these years later, to simply know he was alive would be quite a comfort. I never considered going to my father for help, either—he seemed to not want anything to do with me, let alone an out-of-wedlock grandchild.

That horrible Saturday in September of 1981, Alan once again waited in the car. He informed me that he didn't want to go inside and face a room full of weeping women. I felt his abandonment as I closed the car door behind me, and later I would realize that the anger against my father's similar rejection was triggered then as well. Deep loneliness overwhelmed me as I climbed the stairs to the abortion clinic, but I felt there was no turning back.

I remember my thoughts pivoting in two distinct directions. One side of my heart felt like I should run away and leave this place because I would certainly regret it forever. Another side relayed that this was the best decision I could make. The war between my thoughts made me even more confused, but I gathered my courage, knowing that Alan would abandon me if I didn't follow through with our decision. I believe now that the Holy Spirit was reaching my heart, but I was too scared to listen or comprehend it as a divine message.

The clinic waiting room was filled with weeping women—Alan had been exactly correct. I wondered if he had brought another girlfriend to have an abortion. It didn't matter. I paid the amount required and tried to stay calm. Quickly, my name was called and I was led to another room.

The attendant placed a piece of paper in front of me, instructing me to sign it. "What is it?" I asked. She responded, "It's your counseling."

As I signed the paper, I asked the attendant, "Will this affect me emotionally or psychologically?" I still don't know where that question came from as it flowed out of my mouth; I barely understood the definition of those terms. With a cruel smile, she responded, "Oh, no! It's just a blob of tissue. This will make your life better."

Then I followed her into another room, disrobed completely, donned a hospital gown, and greedily consumed the two Valium offered. Finally, I was ushered into a room where three other women waited quietly.

As the Valium began to take effect, I relaxed and spoke to the woman next to me. She was the mother of two children and didn't want a third. The woman across from me was sobbing quietly. The girl in the corner was no more than twelve years old, staring straight ahead like a zombie.

My name was called first, and I followed the nurse into the room containing four hospital beds. At the end of each bed was a large steel tray of surgical instruments. Fear started mounting in my heart. I hadn't expected to be in an operating room facing surgery! I climbed on the bed in the corner, put my feet in the stirrups, and the nurse said, "Please know that you can hold my hand through this. You didn't pay extra for anesthesia, so this is going to hurt."

Almost immediately there was a masked physician at the bottom of the bed. As I was pushed to a lying position, he performed a brief but brutal exam, announcing, "Seven weeks." The sound from the abortion machine filled the room, and as the instruments entered my body, searing pain enveloped my consciousness.

Instinctively, I began to fight the doctor, and his grip on my thighs tightened. Intense cramping began, and I visualized my uterus being ripped from the inside out. I was screaming, and the attendant covered my mouth to silence me. I felt like I was suffocating, and I kept thinking, *God, please forgive me.* My heart was waiting for Alan to burst through the door and save me, but of course he didn't.

Within several minutes, it was over, and the doctor's grip relaxed. The next day, I would discover handprint bruises on my upper thighs where he held me down. Those bruises took over three weeks to heal, and were a reminder of my choice.

As they led me from the room, the mother of two who didn't want a third was being directed to the second bed. Our eyes locked. I couldn't believe she was going through with the procedure—hadn't she heard my screams? My mouth wanted to warn her, but the pain and agony of the procedure had left me speechless. Our eyes met again, and for an instant I knew she understood my mental warnings—she looked very scared.

As we approached the next room, I heard a strange noise. When we entered, I saw at least twenty women lying on cots, weeping. Later I would recognize the sound as listed in Jeremiah 31:15: "A voice is heard in Ramah, mourning and great weeping, Rachel weeping for her children and refusing to be comforted, because her children are no more." We all knew that we had lost something very precious in the abortion procedure and that our children were no more.

Then I heard the mother of two screaming as they performed her abortion. My heart broke at the sound of her screams, and instinctively I wanted to rescue her. It is one thing to scream yourself and another to lie still while someone else calls out in pain. Then the weeping in the room grew louder and seemed to override her screams.

When I had entered the clinic, I'd felt like my heart was breaking. When I left, I was a completely different person—one part of me was dead and the other part was deeply wounded. With each step down those four flights of stairs, my heart grew colder and harder, stirred with anger to combat my looming pain and grief.

Alan met me at the bottom of the stairs. He picked me up, twirled me around, happy to see me, and said, "Oh, Sydna, I thought they killed you up there." His embrace intensified my physical pain, and I fought him off. He let me go, but I could see that he had been very worried about me.

I couldn't speak, but I thought, *I could have died up there! What other consequences could there be to that abortion?* Then I looked in his face and realized the second truth—*he had thought they were killing me yet waited in the car*. Hatred against him instantly began to build within my heart.

We said little to each other as we got to the car. Like so many other couples, the abortion was rarely discussed, and only in moments of anger. I asked him to pass me a joint; and as the marijuana took effect, the pain began to fade. I tried to fight the hatred, because I needed this man. He was the only one who shared this secret. Alan was also my source of drugs. I remember clearly justifying my medicating actions by saying to myself, *You've done the worst thing possible in taking the life of your firstborn. Why hold back from doing anything else? Nothing you can do now could be worse than the abortion!* That mind-set led me down many other painful and sinful paths.

Going Forward

You may be hurting right now because my story might have dredged up some painful memories of your own story. But I want to encourage you to continue reading, and to not be discouraged by how you're feeling at this moment. Redemption is ahead for you. Your journey to wholeness in Christ might be instantaneous, but more likely it will be a long procession.

Some of you are reading this book because you know or suspect that a loved one could be struggling with this pain and you are unsure how to comfort her. Begin by understanding that she needs your unconditional love and acceptance. There is no sin that God cannot forgive, yet many of us struggle to forgive ourselves for making this decision and sacrificing our own flesh and blood on the altar of choice. Abortion needn't be an unspoken topic around us, but it must be carefully and kindly addressed without condemnation, so as to not bring further guilt and shame to our hearts. Faced with a similar situation, anyone could have made the same choice.

We have all been touched by abortion, whether we know it or not. With each abortion a whole segment of family lineage is lost. Grandparents, siblings—both of the post-abortive individual and the aborted child—spouses and those who had a role in helping us make this choice can struggle with a form of secondary post-abortion syndrome. I hope that this book will be a comfort to those readers as well.

I encourage you to read this book with the hope that recovery is possible and a new life in Christ is available for everyone. In pushing through the pain of this choice, healing and peace will come in His time. Outlined on these pages is the recovery process that begins when we understand and recognize the loss of our child, perhaps name, mourn, and grieve that loss, and accept God's forgiveness. Then we are free to forgive ourselves and continue forward in the hope Christ offered on the cross.

Even in the choice of abortion, there is nothing God cannot use for His own glory and power. He never wastes our pain, remember? Because of God's using my testimony with abortion-minded women and men, many children are now alive. Multitudes of post-abortive women (and men!) are now living restored lives because of the healing God inspired through my child's death. There are few joys like holding a child whom God used you to save. Truly, God can redeem your abortion pain and mold it into a powerful tool of hope for others!

I waited patiently for the LORD;
he turned to me and heard my cry.
He lifted me out of the slimy pit,
out of the mud and mire;
he set my feet on a rock
and gave me a firm place to stand.
He put a new song in my mouth,
a hymn of praise to our God.

—Psalm 40:1–3

Chapter 2

Just What Is Post-Abortion Syndrome?

A voice is heard in Ramah,
mourning and great weeping,
Rachel weeping for her children and
refusing to be comforted,
because her children are no more.
—Jeremiah 31:15

"A woman doesn't want an abortion like she wants an ice-cream cone or a Porsche, but like an animal caught in a trap who gnaws off its own leg," Frederica Mathewes-Green, a positive-life minded feminist who started Feminists for Life, has said.[1]

If you have had an abortion, you know exactly what she means. Abortion is not a procedure most women undergo casually. It is something you are driven to in desperation, when the alternatives seem too awful to contemplate. Yet, ironically, the very act meant to produce relief often produces its own special brand of agony in the long run. In this sense, too, the quote hits home. Though the initial physical pain recedes, the emotional pain of abortion lingers like the phantom pain of an amputated limb. To our hearts, this deep, disturbing sense of unrest and regret is what is meant by the term *post-abortion syndrome*. And that may be all the definition you need.

However, a more technical description is available. According to Dr. Vincent Rue, a psychotherapist who has researched the effects of abortion on post-abortive women for over thirty years, the term post-abortion syndrome, or PAS, refers to a type of post-traumatic stress disorder (PTSD) that is characterized by the chronic or delayed development of symptoms resulting from impacted emotional reactions to the perceived physical and emotional trauma of abortion. In other words, long after the abortion, you may develop an emotional or physical reaction; others may have chronic, continuing reactions to the abortion. He proposes four symptoms of PAS:

(1) exposure to or participation in an abortion experience, i.e., the intentional destruction of one's unborn child, which is perceived as traumatic and beyond the range of usual human experience;

(2) uncontrolled negative re-experiencing of the abortion death event, e.g., flashbacks, nightmares, grief, and anniversary reactions;

(3) unsuccessful attempts to avoid or deny abortion recollections and emotional pain, which result in reduced responsiveness to others and one's environment; and

(4) experiencing associated symptoms not present before the abortion, including guilt about surviving.[2]

This leaves the woman with an inability to,

- process the fear, anger, sadness, and guilt surrounding her abortion experience,
- grieve the loss of her baby, and
- come to peace with God, herself, and others involved in the abortion decision.

Why do so many women experience PAS? After all, most women sincerely believed they were making the best decision they could at the time. The reason probably lies in our creation: God designed mothers to protect their young at all costs. This design is deeply shattered in an abortion decision. And even though abortion is legal, many women feel they have violated their own moral code by choosing it.

Scientific, statistically significant research on post-abortive women has yet to be completed. The scanty research completed by abortion-rights groups cites surveys completed within two years following an abortion without contemplating effects five, ten, twenty, or forty years later. In his recommendation for a longitudinal study to investigate psychological reactions to abortion, former Surgeon General C. Everett Koop raised the concern that 50 percent or more of women who have had an abortion will conceal it from interviewers.[3]

The American Psychological Association recently established a "Task Force on Mental Heath and Abortion" that concluded, "it is clear that some women do experience sadness, grief, and feelings of loss following termination of a pregnancy, and some experience clinically significant disorders, including depression and anxiety."[4]

Because abortion is such a political issue, information related to the potential for regret after abortion is often met with strong opposition. In her article titled "The Mourning After," reporter Sarah Blustain[5] went so far as to say that "PAS is a political strategy masquerading as a psychological crisis."[6] Morgan Winters responded soundly to her point by saying,

> This sounds frighteningly similar to the reasoning behind the dismissal of Post Traumatic Stress Disorder in soldiers coming back from the Vietnam War. The government perceived that acknowledging the disorder would be politically damaging, and it mysteriously went undiagnosed. This famous case of political-medical denial, of course, does not prove the existence of PAS. Yet it does show that just because science hasn't rubber-stamped a condition, doesn't mean people aren't truly suffering. Nor does the political perversion of an issue invalidate the issue itself. All claims, whether they suit one's political inclinations or not, should be taken with a healthy helping of skepticism.[7]

While research has yet to be conducted, the court system in the United States is willing to admit PAS as a possibility. The U.S. Supreme Court, in its closely divided 5-4 ruling in the *Gonzales v. Carhart* decision upholding the first-ever federal ban on an abortion method, ventured into this topic. Oddly, the majority opinion acknowledged the lack of scientific support for post-abortion syndrome while also giving the syndrome some credence. Justice Kennedy's majority opinion said, "[w]hile we find no reliable data to measure the phenomenon, it seems unexceptionable to conclude some women come to regret their choice to abort the infant life they once created and sustained."[8]

As I've said before, women may feel immediate relief, but that is often temporary. Any moral struggle felt prior to the abortion could resurface eventually. Even a woman who had no qualms about abortion at the time may later change her thinking about the issue—perhaps after accepting Christ as her Savior or even just learning more about fetal development—and come to regard with horror the choice she made. Or she may find herself unable to conceive again, and experience profound regret at her lost opportunity for motherhood.

Unable to go back and undo the abortion, the post-abortive woman struggles to cope with the uncomfortable or frightening thoughts and feelings that sometimes plague her. She may try to rationalize her abortion, reminding herself over and over of why she chose it. She may even claim out loud to be glad for what she did, in hopes that if she says it loudly enough and often enough, she may come to believe it inside. She may try to block out the whole experience, pushing it deep inside her heart. Or she may try to make up for the abortion, perhaps working in the pro-life movement, becoming "Super Mom" to her other kids, or having an "atonement baby" soon after the abortion. If she had the abortion for a specific reason, like finishing college or saving a relationship, she may work extremely hard to make that reason valid in retrospect, perhaps becoming heavily invested in making her career a great success, or marrying someone despite reservations.

These defense mechanisms are very effective in keeping the

painful memories at bay, but they consume a lot of mental energy as a woman works to ignore powerful emotions. Eventually, if enough stress enters her life, she may find that she lacks the stamina to cope with both the current stresses and the past ones. During this time, almost anything—pictures of prenatal development, a new pregnancy, or even the whine of a vacuum cleaner or dentist's drill that resembles the sound of the abortionist's equipment—may trigger the symptoms of PAS, which parallel the symptoms of Post Traumatic Stress Disorder, causing her to wonder what is going wrong. She may even question her sanity.

The symptoms of PAS will not necessarily appear at the same time, nor is any woman likely to experience all of them. Some may occur immediately after an abortion, and others much later. However, if three or more of the symptoms listed below describe what you have been going through recently, chances are you are experiencing PAS.[9]

(1) **Guilt.** Guilt is what an individual feels when she has violated her own moral code. For the woman who has come to believe, at some point either before or after the abortion, that she consented to taking the life of her unborn child, the burden of guilt is relentless. In fact, many post-abortive women believe that any unhappy events that have occurred since the abortion were because they "deserve it."

(2) **Anxiety.** Anxiety is defined as an unpleasant emotional and physical state of apprehension that may take the form of tension (inability to relax, irritability), physical responses (dizziness, pounding heart, upset stomach, headaches), worry about the future, difficulty

concentrating, and disturbed sleep. The conflict between a woman's moral standards and her decision to abort generates much of this anxiety. Very often, she will not relate her anxiety to a past abortion, and yet she will unconsciously begin to avoid anything having to do with babies. She may make excuses for not attending a baby shower, skip the baby aisle at the grocery store, and so forth.

(3) **Psychological "numbing."** Many post-abortive women maintain a secret vow that they will never again allow themselves to be put in such a vulnerable position. As a result, often without conscious thought, they may work hard to keep their emotions in tight check, preventing themselves from feeling the pain of what has happened, but also greatly hampering their ability to form and maintain close relationships. Cut off even from themselves, they may feel as though their lives are happening to another person.

(4) **Depression and thoughts of suicide**. All of us experience depression from time to time, but the following forms of it are certainly common in women who have experienced abortion:

- Sad mood—ranging from feelings of melancholy to total hopelessness.
- Sudden and uncontrollable crying episodes—the source of which appear to be a total mystery.
- Deterioration of self-concept—because she feels wholly deficient in her ability to function as a "normal" woman.
- Sleep, appetite, and sexual disturbances—usually in a pattern of insomnia, loss of appetite, and/or reduced sex drive.

- Reduced motivation—for the normal activities of life. The things that occupied her life before the depression no longer seem worth doing.

- Disruption in interpersonal relationships—because of a general lack of enthusiasm for all activities. This is especially evidenced in her relationship with her husband or boyfriend, particularly if he was involved in the abortion decision.

- Thoughts of suicide—or preoccupation with death. Not surprisingly, in a study done by the Elliot Institute, some 33 percent of post-abortive women surveyed reached a level of depression so deep that they would rather die than go on.[10] If you, or someone you know, has verbalized feelings this desperate, you or they are experiencing the severest form of clinical depression. Please get immediate professional attention.

(5) **Anniversary syndrome.** In the same survey, some 54 percent of post-abortive women report an increase of PAS symptoms around the anniversary of the abortion and/or the due date of the aborted child.

(6) **Reexperiencing the abortion.** A very common event described by post-abortive women is the sudden, distressing, recurring flashbacks of the abortion episode. Flashbacks often occur during situations that resemble some aspect of the abortion, such as a routine gynecological exam, or even the sound of a vacuum cleaner's suction. Flashbacks also occur in the form of recurring nightmares about babies in general or

the aborted baby in particular. These dreams usually involve themes of lost, dismembered, or crying babies.

(7) **Preoccupation with becoming pregnant again.** A significant percentage of women who abort become pregnant again within one year, and many others verbalize the desire to conceive again as quickly as possible. The new baby, sometimes referred to as the "atonement child," may represent an unconscious desire to replace the one that was aborted.

(8) **Anxiety over fertility and childbearing issues.** Some post-abortive women maintain a fear that they will never again become pregnant or never be able to carry a pregnancy to term. Some expect to have handicapped children because they have "disqualified themselves as good mothers." Many refer to these fears as punishments from God.

(9) **Interruption of the bonding process with present and/or future children.** Fearing another devastating loss, a post-abortive woman may not allow herself to truly bond with other children. Another common reaction is to atone for her actions toward the aborted child by becoming the world's most perfect mother to her remaining or future children. Likewise, the woman who already had children at the time of her abortion may discover that she is beginning to view them in a different light. At one extreme she may unconsciously devalue them, thinking things like *You were the lucky ones; you were allowed to live.* Or she may go in the opposite direction and become overly protective.

(10) **Survival guilt.** Most women do not abort for trivial reasons. They are usually in the midst of a heartbreaking situation where they stand to lose much if they choose to carry their pregnancies to term. In the end, the decision boils down to a sorrowful "it's me or you, and I choose me." But while the abortion frees them from their current trauma, it frequently produces in them an unrelenting guilt for choosing their own comfort over the life of the child.

(11) **Development of eating disorders.** Some post-abortive women develop anorexia or bulimia. While this phenomenon remains largely unexplored at this time, several factors may contribute to it. First, a substantial weight gain or severe weight loss is associated with unattractiveness, which reduces the odds of becoming pregnant again. Second, becoming unattractive serves as a form of self-punishment and helps perpetuate the belief that the woman is unworthy of anyone's attention. Third, extremes in eating behavior represent a form of control for the woman who feels her life is totally out of control. And finally, a drastic weight loss can shut down the menstrual cycle, thus preventing any future pregnancies.

(12) **Alcohol and drug abuse.** Alcohol and drug use often serve initially as a form of self-medication—a way of coping with the pain of the abortion memories. Sadly, the woman who resorts to alcohol and/or drugs eventually finds herself having not only more problems, but also fewer resources with which to solve them. The mental and physical consequences of alcohol or drug abuse only amplify most of the symptoms the woman is already experiencing.

(13) **Other self-punishing or self-degrading behaviors.** In addition to eating disorders and substance abuse, the post-abortive woman may also enter into abusive relationships, become promiscuous, fail to take care of herself medically, or deliberately hurt herself emotionally and/or physically.

(14) **Brief reactive psychosis.** Rarely, a post-abortive woman may experience a brief psychotic episode for two weeks or less after her abortion. The break with reality and subsequent recovery are both extremely rapid, and in most cases the person returns to normal when it is over. While this is an unusual reaction to abortion, it bears mentioning only because it is possible for a person to have a brief psychotic reaction to a stressful event without being labeled a psychotic individual. During such an episode, the individual's perception of reality is drastically distorted.

While this list of symptoms can be overwhelming, remember that God is the author of all healing. He can wash away each element of pain from your life, restoring you to the peace and security that existed in your heart before making this choice. Take comfort from Isaiah 43:19: "See, I am doing a new thing! Now it springs up; do you not perceive it? I am making a way in the desert and streams in the wasteland." I trust God will use this book to encourage faith that He can heal the desert areas of your heart and pour His streaming love into your soul.

Have mercy on me, O God, have mercy on me,
for in you my soul takes refuge.
I will take refuge in the shadow of your wings
until the disaster has passed.
I cry out to God Most High,
to God, who fulfills his purpose for me.
He sends from heaven and saves me,
rebuking those who hotly pursue me;
God sends his love and faithfulness.

—Psalm 57:1–3

Chapter 3

A Wall of Denial

*I will give you a new heart and put a new spirit
within you; I will take the heart of stone out
of your flesh and give you a heart of flesh.*
—Ezekiel 36:26 NKJV

As I left that clinic, I vowed to distance myself from any of the
memories of that day. In a few short hours, I was a person bent on par-
tying my pain away. My anger was a constant ally in deflecting grief
and was often directed against anyone involved in my abortion choice,
especially Alan. Whenever the memories of my lost child crept toward my
heart, I combated them with drugs and the flimsy excuse that I had only
aborted a blob of tissue. If I was stoned before I went to sleep, there were
no nightmares involving screaming babies. I even avoided infants and
children, as they were dangerous at an emotional level—interacting with

*them seemed to result in depression. I spent some time working for the
abortion rights movement seeking to reinforce that my choice had been a
good one. That experience was short lived because whenever the "a" word
(abortion) was mentioned, my memories of loss resurfaced.*

Denial is a wall of protection that a woman puts up in order to cope
with the reality of her decision. But it is not a difficult wall to erect.
Society provides bricks, mortar, and even laborers for the job.

The wall of denial started during the decision-making process,
just a few bricks at a time, as we began to emotionally detach from
the painful prospect of losing a part of ourselves. A huge section was
raised during the abortion itself, and many bricks have been added
over the years to make the wall taller and stronger. This wall is the
buffer zone of denial to keep us safe from the horrible memories of
losing our children and our own pain in ending their lives.

Unfortunately, the same wall that keeps grief from our heart's
door also keeps us separated from accepting God's redeeming love. It
has been raised to prevent pain and sorrow, but it also acts as a buffer
to other emotions, such as joy and happiness. It may keep us safe, but
it keeps us in prison, too.

C. S. Lewis said,

> To love at all is to be vulnerable. Love anything, and your
> heart will certainly be wrung and possibly be broken. If
> you want to make sure of keeping it intact, you must give
> your heart to no one.... Wrap it carefully round with

hobbies and little luxuries; avoid all entanglements; lock it up safe in the casket or coffin of your selfishness. But in that casket—safe, dark, motionless, airless—it will change. It will not be broken; it will become unbreakable, impenetrable, irredeemable.[1]

By expressing your sorrow over this loss, healing can begin. But before you can begin to break it down, you need to understand the ways in which you fortify it every day.

Denial Under Construction

Two of the bricks, misinformation and the omission of information, can lead a woman to believe the decision to abort is a safe one. The reality is that abortion, like any surgical procedure, brings many risks—psychological, spiritual, emotional, and physical—not only at the time of surgery, but also for future health issues. A report from the Royal College of Psychiatrists in England and Ireland, dated March 2008, stated that, "women should not be allowed to have an abortion until they are counseled on the possible risk to their mental health."

Several studies, including research published in the *Journal of Child Psychology and Psychiatry* in 2006, concluded that abortion in young women might be associated with risks of mental health problems. The controversy intensified when a 2008 inquest in Cornwall, England, heard that a talented artist hanged herself because she was overcome with grief after aborting her twins. Emma Beck, age thirty, left a note saying, "Living is hell for me. I should never have had an abortion. I see now I would have been a good mum. I want to be with my babies; they need me, no one else does."[2]

The "counseling" that many women receive before undergoing an abortion is full of euphemistic terms like "blob of tissue" and "termination of pregnancy." If an ultrasound is done, the screen is normally turned away from the client to avoid her recognizing the unique human aspects of her unborn child. The woman is generally reassured of the legality of abortion, the inference being that anything legal must be okay. She is also comforted with such phrases as "This is the best possible solution for you," and, "A child would only complicate your life, maybe even ruin it. Think about the opportunities you would miss."

Rarely in pro-abortion settings is a woman counseled that she is "taking the life" of her child, or urged to think of anyone but herself, except in such false ways as considering the kind of life the child would have if he or she were rejected by his or her father. This dehumanizing of the baby only fosters the kind of denial that later comes to haunt most women who choose abortion.

Denial-related Bricks

Three more bricks that post-abortive women generally have in abundant supply are guilt, shame, and anxiety. Let's look at each of these up close and see whether they form any part of your wall.

Guilt

We hear a lot about guilt these days. We're reassured over and over of God's forgiveness and are encouraged to give ourselves room to fail. This is all well and good. Feelings of guilt that occur when you've done nothing wrong, or that linger after forgiveness has been granted—these are false guilt, and they should be put aside.

But true guilt is another matter. When you have broken one of God's laws, true guilt results. While we may not have looked at our abortion as a sin at the time, it was one just the same. God makes it very clear in Scripture that He is the author of all life:

> I will praise You, for I am fearfully and wonderfully made;
>> Marvelous are Your works,
>> And that my soul knows very well.
> My frame was not hidden from You,
>> When I was made in secret,
>> And skillfully wrought in the lowest parts of the earth.
> Your eyes saw my substance, being yet unformed.
>> And in Your book they all were written,
>> The days fashioned for me,
>> When as yet there were none of them.
> (Ps. 139:14–16 NKJV)

We played God's role by ending our children's lives in an effort to erase our mistake and hide it from the world. Guilty feelings probably played a role in your having an abortion in the first place … guilt over what an unplanned pregnancy would do to your family, to your boyfriend, even to the baby itself. Yet the very act that was supposed to alleviate that guilt only produced guilt of a different sort—true guilt before God.

But there is wonderful news. You don't have to live with that guilt forever; it can be forgiven! First John 1:9 (NKJV) tells us: "If we confess our sins, He is faithful and just to forgive us our sins and to cleanse us from all unrighteousness."

This truth brings the realization that the secret of abortion lives and thrives in darkness, denial, and with deceit from the Enemy. Bringing the truth to the light takes away the power of the Enemy and gives it to the Lord. In His light this past choice is cleansed, healed, and can no longer fester and grow, as outlined in Luke 12:3: "What you have said in the dark will be heard in the daylight, and what you have whispered in the ear in the inner rooms will be proclaimed from the roofs."

God can remove the awful gnawing of that guilt from our souls, and what's more, He longs to do it! But the more you try to escape that guilt in other ways, the more bricks you add to your wall—and the more you seal yourself off from a thriving relationship with God, as well as from truly experiencing the joys of life.

One psalmist described the feelings of ignored guilt this way:

> When I kept silent, my bones grew old through my groaning all the day long. For day and night Your hand was heavy upon me; my vitality was turned into the drought of summer. (Ps. 32:3–4 NKJV).

The way to receive relief from guilt is to acknowledge your sins to God in the privacy of your heart. Remember that God knows everything—including the truth about your abortion. You are not telling Him anything He doesn't already know. Trust Him with your heart and let the wall fall down. You'll be amazed at the view on the other side, just as David wrote:

> I acknowledged my sin to You,
>   And my iniquity I have not hidden.

I said, "I will confess my transgressions to the LORD,"
And You forgave the iniquity of my sin.
(Ps. 32:5 NKJV)

In his *Old Testament Commentary*, Warren Wiersbe outlines the following points about this passage of Scripture:

> This is the second of the seven penitential psalms. David wrote it after confessing to God his sins of adultery, murder, and deception. This psalm ... is a part of the fulfillment of [David's] promise [to share what he'd learned from this costly experience]. David offered no excuses; he admitted that he had sinned and was guilty before God.
>
> Guilt is to the conscience what pain is to the body: it tells us that something is wrong and must be made right, or things will get worse.... But God's forgiveness isn't a negative thing; the Lord adds positive blessings to help us on the road to recovery. David exchanged hiding his sins for a hiding place in the Lord. God removed his troubles and put a wall of protection around him.
>
> Did David deserve those blessings? Of course not, nor do we! But this is the grace of God as found in Jesus Christ our Lord. This doesn't mean that David didn't suffer because of the consequences of his sins. God in his grace forgives us, but God in his government says, "You shall reap what you have sown."[3]

Shame

Another common brick in the post-abortive heart is shame. Satan continually whispers in our ears the lie that if people knew about this choice, they would hate us.

In an effort to protect yourself from this potential rejection, you may hide the abortion from those around you. Or you may go to the opposite extreme and tell everyone around you, driven by your hunger to have them answer the question, "Will you still love me if you know the truth?"

Sometimes the thoughts of unworthiness flooded my mind until I thought I would scream. I kept hearing the words, "You're not worthy of anything good. You don't deserve forgiveness. How could you have taken the life of your own child? You deserve anything bad that happens to you, and worse." I couldn't sleep without being high because of the thoughts that raced inside my head, leading from one scenario of doom and gloom to another. Instead of confiding in someone trustworthy about these battles that raged on in my head, I kept them locked up inside me, too ashamed to admit my struggle to anyone, feeling like I was certainly going crazy.

At one point about two months after the abortion, I wanted to leave Alan. He was a reminder of the abortion, and we weren't getting along very well. Our relationship had deteriorated significantly—I'm sure I was a reminder to him of that difficult day also. On a weekend trip for a class I was taking, I met another student, a man who immediately showed interest. He was kind, and I knew before too long that he was interested in me. When we arrived at our destination and I lay down to sleep, I let my mind linger over this new man. Then I was overcome with fear at the possibility that this man may not be able to love someone who had chosen abortion. Immediately my walls went up, and I cut off his attention the next day. He was obviously disappointed but didn't pursue me further. I would never know if my fears over his possible rejection were justified. I never gave him the opportunity to be a good guy.

Several months later I was at an off-campus party with Alan. This man came to the party and sat across the room, looking at me intently. Alan noticed the look and saw my returned smile. He angrily pulled me out of the apartment and said, "He's interested in you, isn't he?" I objected, but Alan then put into words what my heart had already warned me. "If you are thinking about leaving me for him, keep in mind that I'll be sure to tell him about your abortion. He'd never want you if he knew about that!" Thinking that Alan was correct, I never gave this man a chance. The shame of my abortion was often a weapon Alan used to keep me bound to him.

The *American Heritage Dictionary* defines *shame* as "a painful emotion caused by a strong sense of guilt, embarrassment, unworthiness, or disgrace."[4] But any woman who has had an abortion doesn't need a dictionary to tell her about shame. She could write a dictionary on it herself.

Psalm 25:3 (NKJV) tells us, "Indeed, let no one who waits on You [God] be ashamed; let those be ashamed who deal treacherously without cause." When you seek the Lord, confess your sins, and ask Him to forgive you, you are released from shame. Psalm 34:4–5 (NKJV) relays this truth:

> I sought the LORD, and He heard me,
>> And delivered me from all my fears.
> They looked to Him and were radiant,
>> And their faces were not ashamed.

You will likely be surprised by the grace in people's reactions to your long-held secret; the condemning few are mostly just on television. When I share my abortion story with large crowds, I see the faces of women and men who are most likely post-abortive. Later they've quietly told me that my story is just like theirs. They express shock at how the audience received me with compassion. It has proved to them that their secret is not too dark to share. Many husbands also have thanked me because I outlined their wife's abortion experience and allowed them to understand her pain at a deeper level. Most men wonder about this event but are afraid to ask for details. But no matter what anyone else thinks, once you confess your sin to God, your shame will begin to evaporate.

Anxiety

Your wall doesn't have to crumble much before anxiety begins to pour in. Any thought of the aborted baby as a real child, and the questions will begin: *Was it a boy or a girl? Who would he or she have looked like? What would we be doing now if I had kept her?*

Seeing a baby or a child/teen/adult who would be about the same age as your aborted child can trigger the anxiety. *Is that what he'd look like? I wonder if her hair would have been like that.* Every time one of those questions is asked, you have forced yourself to set it aside, thinking you can't dwell on such thoughts because they are too painful.

You may never know the answers to these questions on earth, and that unknowingness makes you vulnerable to anguish and despair. Each time you put off thinking about your child as a human being, you add another brick to your wall. In a manner of speaking, your lost child will continue to haunt your heart until he or she is recognized there. It's time to begin to process these thoughts and realize that they will not hurt you, but heal you as you let your child become a part of your life.

People in Denial

Denial is not new with the legalization of abortion. It's not even new to the twentieth century. In fact, the Bible is full of examples of people in denial—not just to God and others, but to themselves.

Eve's Story (Gen. 3:2–20)

Ironically, the first denial story involves the very first woman—Eve, in the Garden of Eden. It's a familiar tale. Adam and Eve are given the run of the garden, except for one tree, which is forbidden to them. Satan, disguised as a snake, tempts Eve to eat the fruit of that tree, and she succumbs, convincing Adam to go along. When confronted by God, she turns the blame onto the snake.

How many of us, after our abortions, began to support the pro-abortion movement? Like Eve recruiting Adam, did we need company in our wrongdoing to make it feel acceptable? Finding acceptance can add a powerful brick to our wall of denial. And like Eve when God confronted her, how many of us blamed others for their bad advice or lack of support, instead of assuming the responsibility for our own actions?

Just as Eve was deceived into believing that the forbidden fruit would make her smarter, many women today are deceived into believing that an unplanned pregnancy will ruin their lives. They are mistaken—just as Eve was.

David's Story (2 Samuel 11)

Even one of the heroes of the Bible, David, tried to hide from his sin—a sin, incidentally, much like ours.

Bathsheba, a lovely young woman, was bathing on a rooftop, and David caught sight of her. Quite naturally aroused, he decided to act on his desire, and he had her brought to him. The result of his passion was a pregnancy, his child conceived in the womb of another man's wife.

David first tried to cover up his actions by bringing her soldier-husband, Uriah, home from battle in the hopes that Uriah would lie with her and then assume that the child was his own. When this plan didn't work, David had Uriah sent to the front lines, knowing he would be killed and that Bathsheba would then be free to marry David, thus legitimizing the pregnancy.

Deception, manipulation, justification, even murder ... all to avoid being found out through the truth of an unplanned pregnancy. Was it any different with our abortions? In our panic, we added more bricks to the wall. Weren't we willing to go to any lengths rather than face our friends or family with the truth, risking rejection and judgment, possibly losing our reputation, our lifestyle, and the opportunities we'd anticipated?

Peter's Story (Luke 22:54–62)

Imagine knowing Jesus as a flesh-and-blood human being. Imagine being selected as His special disciple, walking with Him by the Sea of Galilee, watching His miracles in amazement and listening in awe to

His teachings. How could you experience Christ face-to-face and not be completely loyal to Him? Yet that's what happened to Peter.

One minute he was declaring his absolute loyalty to the Savior; the next, he was abandoning Him in His time of greatest need. The soldiers had taken Jesus away to be tried and crucified. Peter followed and was recognized as one of His friends. But when asked if he knew Jesus, he denied it on three occasions.

His denial, of course, stemmed from his fear of receiving the same treatment Jesus was getting. But as Jesus predicted, when Peter heard the rooster crow, he realized he had denied the Lord three times, and his wall of denial crumbled in a torrent of weeping as he begged for forgiveness.

Denial Within You

Have you built a wall of denial? If so, try to reconstruct the process through which you convinced yourself that your abortion was a good decision. The following questions may help:

- What were your fears at the time of the abortion?
- What pressures did you experience, and from whom?
- What was your understanding of abortion, and how did you gain this understanding? You may not even have recognized the wall of denial being built in your life. If you believed all the misinformation and lies that were told, then you may have thought it truly was a good choice for you at the time. But since abortion is a legitimate loss, your subconscious may have responded for you. You may not have understood the post-abortion syndrome thoughts

and behaviors at the time, but you are just beginning to understand them now.

Below is a list of some of the arguments commonly used to build and keep the wall of denial firmly in place. Do some of them represent the bricks in your own wall?

- *I only terminated a pregnancy; I didn't lose a baby.*
- *Abortion is now safe and legal. Millions choose it with no obvious consequences. How can it be wrong?*
- *Everyone has a different perspective as to when life begins.*
- *It happened so long ago; why bring it up now?*
- *Everyone around me said it would be the best thing to do.*

Jesus has said that the truth, His truth, will make us free (John 8:32) and part of that encompasses freedom from denial, living a lie. Just as we have built our walls of denial brick by brick, we must begin the work of tearing them down brick by brick with the truth. Are you ready to begin the work? If so, take a quiet moment to tear down the lies and replace them with the truth. Maybe even writing these words down will help you solidify them in your heart and mind.

I only terminated a pregnancy; I didn't lose a baby.

> For You formed my inward parts;
> > You covered me in my mother's womb.
> I will praise You, for I am fearfully and wonderfully made;

> Marvelous are Your works,
> And that my soul knows very well.
> My frame was not hidden from You,
> When I was made in secret,
> And skillfully wrought in the lowest parts of the earth.
> Your eyes saw my substance, being yet unformed.
> And in Your book they all were written,
> The days fashioned for me,
> When as yet there were none of them.
> (Ps. 139:13–16 NKJV)

Abortion is now safe and legal. Millions choose it with no obvious consequences. How can it be wrong?

> There is a way that seems right to a man, But its end is the way of death. (Prov. 14:12 NKJV)

Everyone has a different perspective as to when life begins.

> Where is the wise? Where is the scribe? Where is the disputer of this age? Has not God made foolish the wisdom of this world? (1 Cor. 1:20 NKJV)

It happened so long ago; why bring it up now?

> And there is no creature hidden from His sight, but all things are naked and open to the eyes of Him to whom we must give account. (Heb. 4:13 NKJV)

Everyone around me said it would be the best thing to do.

> For do I now persuade men, or God? Or do I seek to
> please men? For if I still pleased men, I would not be a
> bondservant of Christ. (Gal. 1:10 NKJV)

In his testimony before a congressional committee, Dr. C. Ever-ett Koop, former Surgeon General of the United States, stated the obvious: "The consequences to the fetus [in abortion] are undeni-able."[5] In your heart, you know this. But what the heart knows, the mind sometimes has trouble accepting. Yet before you can begin to heal, you will have to acknowledge consciously the truth of what you have done—that your decision to abort ended the life of your unborn child.

How can you begin to tear down your wall of denial? Facing the truth that abortion ended a life is the first step in grieving, allowing us to understand that our emotions following our abortion are in response to our losing a child.

My husband, Tom, and I struggled with infertility in our early years of marriage. I was always scared that my abortion would affect my ability to get pregnant. Through a series of tests, my doctor came to the conclusion that the abortion had been incomplete and my tubes were blocked. Once he cleared those tubes, I became pregnant quickly. Even pregnant, I was hesitant and scared, wondering if God would allow me to actually become a mother of a living child.

Denial was a common tool to help me distance myself from the haunting memories of the tiny being that I lost on the day of my abortion. The pregnancy was a constant reminder of my lost child.

I was sixteen weeks along when a sudden and jabbing pain hit my abdomen. I ran to the bathroom and discovered I was hemorrhaging. In that fearful moment, I got down on my hands and knees and cried out to the Lord, begging Him to forgive me for the abortion and to spare the life of my unborn son. Within fifteen minutes, Tom had me in the doctor's office, where we heard Bruce's heartbeat and the hemorrhaging stopped. I thanked the Lord, knowing He had intervened. But there was a consequence to my confession—God took control of my heart once again. Five minutes later an ultrasound revealed Bruce for the first time, dancing in my womb and sucking his thumb. I'd expected to see a blob of tissue. I finally knew the truth. I hadn't aborted a blob of tissue—but a baby. After that, I would never again be successful in denying the humanity of my aborted child.

For you, that moment may not have come. Perhaps now is the time to take out all the memories you have worked so hard to suppress, open the door to that closet in your mind where those dark scrapbooks are hidden.

It's time to clean house. But it won't be easy. Facing our mistakes never is, and this one is likely to bring a depth of grief and regret unparalleled so far in your life. It would be a good idea to join a recovery class as you go through this, or at least confide in a supportive friend. However, in releasing the denial, you will find once again a measure of relief. For in acknowledging the truth, you will be giving yourself the opportunity to mourn consciously what you have been grieving subconsciously all along—the death of your own child.

God's Response to Your Abortion

One of the hardest things about bringing your sin into the light is the realization that, not only can you see it, but God can too. It may be comforting to remember that, to Him, your abortion has never been hidden. He knew your baby before you even knew of his or her existence. He has always known the circumstances of his or her conception. He was with your child as it was being formed in your womb, and He was present when your baby died. And He is with your child even now.

He is with you, as He was with Eve, and with David, and with Peter.

He knew of all your turmoil way back then. He knew what you thought. He knew what you had been told, what pressures you were under, what fears you faced, and what cowardice or temptations won you over. He loved you then, and He still loves you now. His love will never end.

You mustered up the courage to enter the abortion clinic that day; now summon that courage back again, this time to call on the Lord. He can free you from the guilt of this sin. Stop now and ask Him to reveal to you the things your mind has hidden from conscious thought since the abortion. Remembering is the first step in tearing down the wall of denial. Trust that He will not burden you with more than your heart can bear. It's a painful step, but it is the first one on the road to real relief … a relief that will last.

Consider these other passages that speak about darkness and light, and have hope …

John 12:35–36 (NKJV) Then Jesus said to them, "A little while longer the light is with you. Walk while you have the light, lest darkness overtake you; he who walks in darkness does not know where he is going. While you have the light, believe in the light, that you may become sons of light." These things Jesus spoke, and departed, and was hidden from them.

Romans 13:12 (NKJV) The night is far spent, the day is at hand. Therefore let us cast off the works of darkness, and let us put on the armor of light.

John 3:19–21 (NKJV) And this is the condemnation, that the light has come into the world, and men loved darkness rather than light, because their deeds were evil. For everyone practicing evil hates the light and does not come to the light, lest his deeds should be exposed. But he who does the truth comes to the light, that his deeds may be clearly seen, that they have been done in God.

Ephesians 6:12–15 For our struggle is not against flesh and blood, but against the rulers, against the authorities, against the powers of this dark world and against the spiritual forces of evil in the heavenly realms. Therefore put on the full armor of God, so that when the day of evil comes, you may be able to stand your ground, and after you have done everything, to stand. Stand firm then, with the belt of truth buckled around your waist, with the breastplate of righteousness in place, and with your feet fitted with the readiness that comes from the gospel of peace.

1 Peter 2:9 But you are a chosen generation, a royal priesthood, a holy nation, His own special people, that you may proclaim the praises of Him who called you out of darkness into His marvelous light.

As you allow these scriptures to penetrate your heart's walls, know that God will be with you at each step of the way. He will reconstruct these memories, heal the devastation that your abortion caused, and bring you safely through to a place of restoration. All you have to do is ask Him for His help.

....

Create in me a pure heart, O God,
and renew a steadfast spirit within me.
Do not cast me from your presence
or take your Holy Spirit from me.
Restore to me the joy of your salvation
and grant me a willing spirit, to sustain me.
Then I will teach transgressors your ways,
and sinners will turn back to you.
Save me from bloodguilt, O God,
the God who saves me,
and my tongue will sing of your righteousness.
O Lord, open my lips,
and my mouth will declare your praise . . .
The sacrifices of God are a broken spirit;
a broken and contrite heart,
O God, you will not despise.
          —Psalm 51:10–17

....

Chapter 4

Bitter Roots: Anger

*... that no bitter root grows up to
cause trouble and defile many.*
—Hebrews 12:15

Whenever I heard the word abortion *my heart would grow angry. In the first years, that anger was directed against the pro-life movement, which, in my mind, would certainly have judged me. There was always anger against my mother, whom I continued to blame for not being emotionally stable enough for me to come to her with the truth of my pregnancy. While trying to get pregnant with my first son, and going through fertility issues that were possibly connected to the abortion, that anger turned toward the individuals who had worked at the abortion clinic. When I saw my son on the ultrasound screen, that anger turned against myself and rested there until God's peace finally broke through.*

Emotions play a pivotal role in the event of a crisis. They become the avenue by which we vent our feelings of anger and pain, sadness and remorse. When we don't allow those emotions to play their important role in the process of healing at the time of the event, they will resurface in the future.[1]

One of the strongest of human passions, anger, seldom leaves us without being addressed directly. When denied, it finds other ways to express itself, often through bitterness or depression. Yet when it is expressed inappropriately, it can be terribly destructive to anyone unfortunate enough to be in its path.

Signs of "aftershock," a word coined by Dr. Andrew Scaby to describe any significant delayed response to a crisis,[2] may vary from sleep disturbances, jumpiness, nightmares, guilt, and numbness. Dr. Anne C. Speckhard, in a survey of post-abortive women, found that 92 percent of those surveyed reported feelings of anger related to their abortions, and most of them expressed surprise at the intensity of those feelings.[3] Unsure how to handle it, many worked hard to keep that anger in check, succeeding only in driving it underground to seethe and fester and express itself in other ways. Many women find themselves having spontaneous, emotional outbursts triggered by the least provocation. They can't seem to control their emotions or figure out where they are coming from, which is as confusing for the individual as it is to those closest to her.

Whether it seethes on the surface or hides underneath, anger is an emotion that needs attention. When it's related to abortion, it often acts as a roadblock to healing—around which there is no detour. The good news is that it's an emotion familiar to our heavenly Father. And with His help we can find a healthy way of handling it.

Anger in the Bible

We tend to think of anger as a negative quality, something that demands our repentance, which is certainly the case many times. Yet it's a quality God Himself bestowed upon humanity. In fact, it's a quality He possesses.

God's Anger

It's not hard at all to find biblical examples of God getting angry. Old Testament pages flow with it! Psalm 78:49–50 (NKJV) gives a graphic description of His attitude toward the Egyptians, who had enslaved the Israelites:

> He cast on them the fierceness of His anger,
> Wrath, indignation, and trouble,
> By sending angels of destruction among them.
> He made a path for His anger;
> He did not spare their soul from death,
> But gave their life over to the plague.

The story of God's anger against Sodom and Gomorrah in Genesis 19:1–20 is a familiar one. Because of the wickedness of the people of Sodom, God rained fire and brimstone upon the entire city, killing all who lived there. A quick glance through a concordance gives us many more instances when God's wrath was displayed.

Not only does God allow anger, He also encourages it—but only when it's directed against evil. Much of the anger related to your abortion undoubtedly qualifies.

Jesus' Anger

Few who have ever attended Sunday school could have missed the story of Jesus' anger toward the moneychangers in the temple. Like Father, like Son—He was outraged to have this holy place used like a common flea market, for selfish profit, distracting those who had come to worship. John 2:13–16 (NKJV) tells the story:

> Now the Passover of the Jews was at hand, and Jesus went up to Jerusalem. And He found in the temple those who sold oxen and sheep and doves, and the moneychangers doing business. When He had made a whip of cords, He drove them all out of the temple, with the sheep and the oxen, and poured out the changers' money and overturned the tables. And He said to those who sold doves, "Take these things away! Do not make My Father's house a house of merchandise!"

Hardly a calm reaction! There's not a thing wrong with the emotion of anger, even intense anger; in fact, there's a lot right with it.

Our Anger

We know from experience, however, that anger can be used destructively, hurting both people and relationships. It can be misused in two ways. First, it can be misused when it arises from selfish indignation rather than righteous indignation. For instance, Jesus' anger toward the moneychangers was righteous—they were behaving inappropriately in a place of worship. Now, had He been angry because He had planned to sell doves as well and they had cheated Him out of the best location ... that would have been anger for nothing but self-serving purposes.

The second way anger can be misused is in its expression. Notice that Jesus drove out the right people, the moneychangers. He addressed their behavior, not their beings. How often have we found ourselves exploding at our children for leaving their beds unmade or clothes on the floor, when the real source of our anger is something else entirely? And how many times, when hurt or offended, have we found ourselves calling people names and hurling insults? These are the times when the expression of our anger crosses the line into sin's territory.

Digging Up the Bitter Roots

Have you driven angry feelings so far down inside that they have sprung up as plants with different names, like depression or despair, or perhaps self-destructive behaviors? It's critical that you dig out those tough roots. They are like weeds in your garden: persistent, pervasive, and fully capable of choking out any good seeds you may plant there. You may need to do some emotional probing to find out the true source of those feelings. Ask God to help you see any areas of bitterness or resentment that have remained in your heart. The following list of common targets of post-abortive anger may help:

- People who withheld the truth about the procedure
- Friends who urged abortion as the best option
- Self, for being in the situation to begin with, and for not having enough courage to go through with the pregnancy
- Self, for not educating yourself about contraception, fetal development, and abortion techniques

- The father of the baby, for not being supportive, whether physically, emotionally, or financially, or simply for not proposing marriage
- Society, for offering abortion as a safe solution
- Parents, for pressuring the situation, knowingly or unknowingly, or even insisting on your abortion
- God, for allowing the pregnancy to happen or for not intervening to stop the abortion
- Abortion protestors who may have branded you with malicious and judgmental words

Lack of Anger

Sometimes we have trouble getting angry. We have conditioned our hearts and minds to such an extent that we remain frozen, experiencing neither anger nor joy.

Anger was a forbidden emotion in my heart. My mother had been raised in a physically abusive environment. When she grew up, she vowed no one would yell at her again. Whenever I got angry as a child and raised my voice, my mother would explode. I believe that indirectly my anger triggered her unresolved emotions toward her mother. Her explosions conditioned me to never reveal my anger. When I got married, my husband had to force me to get angry with him, knowing it was unhealthy to hold these emotions inside. Yet it took too much energy to get mad. All that energy was subconsciously focused on keeping away the looming pain over my lost child.

It wasn't until we addressed anger in my post-abortion recovery class that I started to feel the burning sensation of this emotion. I was angry at everyone. It had always been there; I just had never allowed myself to express it. I was angry at my boyfriend for not loving our unborn child; at my mother for not being emotionally strong enough to face another possible scandal; at the university for having the expulsion policy for pregnant unwed students; at the abortion clinic and family planning personnel who never suggested a life choice; and then, finally toward the younger version of myself who had allowed such a thing to happen to my unborn child.

Once you've identified the source—or more likely, sources—of your anger, you'll notice that some of them will be legitimate and others will not. However, there is still a need for these emotions to be expressed in some way to expel the bitterness in your heart. Emotions are not always balanced, but our responses to them certainly can be rational.

Begin by praying that God will direct you in how to address your angry feelings. Most of them can probably be dealt with in the privacy of your own heart, but there may be some that will necessitate your sharing with another person for godly insight. Be slow to do that. Remember, you are uncovering hurts that scabbed over long ago. To you, the words may feel new and raw all over again, and it may take some time to gain perspective on them.

Someone once said that holding on to anger and bitterness is like drinking poison and hoping the other person dies. These emotions hurt our hearts the most. We must address our emotions of anger to begin the process of forgiveness.

✳

It was a simple "time-line" activity that rooted out the major source of anger in my heart many years after I had received healing from my abortion. The time-line process was to list out both the good and bad events in your life, ranking them on a scale of -1 to -10 (bad) and +1 to +10 (good). The activity suggested that we write down what immediately came to mind. I wrote down my parents' divorce as being the worst thing that had ever happened to me. Once it was written I stopped and questioned myself. Could it be that my parents' divorce was worse than my abortion experience? Suddenly I felt a deep level of anger toward my father that I had never realized before.

Like a powder keg, the simple activity unleashed all the hidden recollection of the scandal that haunted my heart. I relived the humility of that small town society that snubbed us for the scandal. I felt the abandonment of my father each and every time he came to pick me up for brief visits. I envisioned Mac's loving face at all my school and church events and my wishing my own father had cared enough to attend.

Why had I not realized before that my father's abandonment was the first leg on my journey that led to an abortion? I was always searching for his love and attention. With that realization, God told me there was more work to be done in my heart. Within a few months, I traveled back to that small town to visually relive those memories, asking God to help me address the anger and contempt that still resided in my heart. He was faithful, and at the end of that journey, I released this long root of anger and felt His peace allowing me to love my birth father again, despite the fact that he may never openly acknowledge his part in my destructive decisions.

A good way to begin to address unresolved anger is to write letters that you **never** intend to send. Pour out all your feelings of rage, betrayal, hurt, or disillusionment onto paper or on a computer screen. Then destroy the documents. Another way is to speak these emotions privately in front of a mirror or walk back through the area where the memories occurred. If they need further expression, do it with a trusted friend or counselor. As time eases the intensity, pray and ask the Lord whether to address the issues with the people who were involved in the abortion decision. If that is His leading, He will help you do that in a loving way.

Bear in mind that God will take vengeance on those who have hurt you, if it is necessary. Romans 12:19 says, "Do not take revenge, my friends, but leave room for God's wrath, for it is written: 'It is mine to avenge; I will repay,' says the Lord." There will be a day in heaven when all of us will account for our lives here on earth.[4]

Do not fret because of evil men
or be envious of those who do wrong;
for like the grass they will soon wither,
like green plants they will soon die away.
Trust in the LORD and do good;
dwell in the land and enjoy safe pasture.
Delight yourself in the LORD
and he will give you the desires of your heart.
Commit your way to the LORD;

trust in him and he will do this:
He will make your righteousness shine like the dawn,
the justice of your cause like the noonday sun.
Be still before the LORD and wait patiently for him;
do not fret when men succeed in their ways,
when they carry out their wicked schemes.
Refrain from anger and turn from wrath;
do not fret—it leads only to evil.

—Psalm 37:1–8

Chapter 5

The Heart of the Matter: Forgiveness

*Those who sat in darkness and in the shadow of
death, bound in affliction and irons—because they
rebelled against the words of God, and despised the
counsel of the Most High, therefore He brought down
their heart with labor; they fell down, and there was
none to help. Then they cried out to the LORD in their
trouble, and He saved them out of their distresses.
He brought them out of darkness and the shadow
of death, and broke their chains in pieces. Oh, that
men would give thanks to the LORD for His goodness,
and for His wonderful works to the children of men!*
—*Psalm 107:10–15 (NKJV)*

I was angry at my mother for being emotionally weak. If I had been able to confide in her, maybe my baby would still be alive. In my torn mind, she was responsible for my son's death even though she never knew I was pregnant.

Forgiveness. In all of Christianity, probably no concept is more familiar; after all, our very salvation depends upon God's forgiveness of our sins. Yet for all its familiarity, forgiveness is probably the aspect of Christianity people wrestle with most deeply. Some of us find it hard to believe God has really forgiven our sins. Others of us just can't forgive ourselves. And we've all struggled with forgiving others.

If you've had an abortion, forgiveness is likely a word you can't hear without feeling as though a strong band has been clenched around your heart. The issues surrounding that topic are probably numerous and conflicting. Simultaneously you may have emotions of guilt, resentment, bitterness, shame, anger, and hopelessness … just to name a few. There is so much to sort out and seemingly no good way to go about it. It may seem easier just to jam those feelings back in, to not think about them.

But forgiveness—from God, toward yourself, and toward others—is essential to the process of healing. It's part of the great gift God longs to give you. It's the key to the spiritual and emotional freedom that is available, just around the corner.

There are ways to sort out the tangled strands that bind your heart. It is possible to release the resentment, to reconcile relationships, to find forgiveness.

Forgiveness from God

At the time, I couldn't imagine that God would forgive my sin of my abortion. Even now, it's still hard to understand that He didn't want me to experience the pain that resulted after my choice; that He wanted to heal my heart and bring me to a place of wholeness. Because of my earthly father's example, thinking of God like a father only made God seem even more distant. It wasn't until I started attending my post-abortion recovery class that I realized that God is nothing like an earthly father because He isn't human!

The grief and pain I was feeling about my abortion wasn't His punishment but His remedy to my heartbreak. He knew that my human body needed to grieve the child I had never held. It was my humanness that I was trying to escape in justifying my abortion. I hated myself and felt I deserved punishment from God, but that wasn't His perspective. It was the voice of the accuser, Satan, who convinced me that God hated me for my sins. The point where my perspective changed was when I gave up and begged for God's forgiveness, and He came much closer than He had ever been before.

The foundational issue to address is forgiveness from God. If you haven't found forgiveness in Him, you will never find lasting peace. It simply isn't available from any other source.

For some of you, that statement drains you of hope. How, you wonder, could God possibly forgive me? How could I even face Him with this? How could I even dare to ask?

If those are your thoughts, they are not coming from God as He
expresses Himself through His Word. What the Bible does offer is a
portrait—in fact, a gallery of portraits, page after page of them—of
your Father's open arms, of His compassionate face, all with captions
affirming in strong language that there is no sin greater than His
capacity to forgive. Take a look at a few of them:

> You are forgiving and good, O Lord, abounding in love
> to all who call to you. (Ps. 86:5)

> Praise the LORD, O my soul, and forget not all his
> benefits—who forgives all your sins and heals all your
> diseases, who redeems your life from the pit and crowns
> you with love and compassion. (Ps. 103:2–4)

> Who is a God like you, who pardons sin and forgives
> the transgression …? You do not stay angry forever but
> delight to show mercy. You will again have compassion
> on us; you will tread our sins underfoot and hurl all our
> iniquities into the depths of the sea. (Mic. 7:18–19)

> Repent, then, and turn to God, so that your sins may be
> wiped out, that times of refreshing may come from the
> Lord, and that he may send the Christ, who has been
> appointed for you—even Jesus. (Acts 3:19–20)

> "Come now, let us reason together," says the LORD.
> Though your sins are like scarlet, they shall be as white as

snow; though they are red as crimson, they shall be like wool. (Isa. 1:18)

If we confess our sins, he is faithful and just and will forgive us our sins and purify us from all unrighteousness. (1 John 1:9)

God's forgiveness hinges on only one thing: our acknowledgment of our own sin. What often keeps us from it? Fear. Look at your other relationships. Maybe you have found it too hard to tell certain people in your life about your abortion. Perhaps it has been your mother's disappointment that you find difficult to face. Maybe it's the look of betrayal on your husband's face that you can't bear to see. Maybe you're afraid of the reaction of your friends if they were ever to find out.

With God, however, there needn't be any fear for two important reasons. First, He already knows about your abortion. You can't shock or surprise Him. He not only knows what you did, but He was there when it happened.

Yes, you read that right.

When you conceived that child, He was there.

When you discovered you were pregnant, He was there.

When you tossed and turned, cried and prayed, panicked and planned, He was there. Did you hear His voice? Did your fear drown it out? Did you close your ears? He knows that too. He knows the worst and the most pitiable about those awful days. He knew even then what you would decide and yet He stayed. His love for you continued.

When you entered the abortion clinic, as you lay on that table, your boyfriend may have been in the car, your mother may have been in the waiting room, but He was there, all the time. With you. With your baby. This is confirmed by Psalm 139:8: "If I go up to the heavens, you are there; if I make my bed in the depths, you are there."

There is nothing you have done that He doesn't know, didn't see. He waits only for you to acknowledge it. But you can do so without fear, because of the second difference: You know His response.

You can't be sure how your friends or your husband or your mother will react. But you can be sure how God will react. He will forgive. He will rejoice. He'll throw a party, and invite all the angels! If you don't believe it, read the story of the prodigal son in Luke 15:11–24: "'For this son of mine was dead and is alive again; he was lost and is found.' So they began to celebrate."

Don't forget, God is used to sinners, as Romans 3:23 says: "For all have sinned and fall short of the glory of God." He hasn't turned one away yet.

Unpardonable Sin

Many post-abortive women read Mark 3:28–29 with great apprehension. This passages says, "I tell you the truth, all the sins and blasphemies of men will be forgiven them. But whoever blasphemes against the Holy Spirit will never be forgiven; he is guilty of an eternal sin." Please understand that simply by wanting to be forgiven and being willing to repent is clear proof that you have not committed the unpardonable sin. This passage relates to the person who has no conscience, and who has hardened his or her heart against the knowledge and need for God's forgiveness. By even choosing to read this book, and being open to the direction of the Holy Spirit in your heart, you have provided evidence that you are not blaspheming the Holy Spirit. Understand that God knows your heart and can discern His Holy Spirit working within you, even when you cannot.

Forgiving Ourselves

The parable of the unforgiving servant in Matthew 18:22–40 is what the Lord used to help me forgive myself. In this passage, one man is brought before the king because he has an unpaid bill of ten thousand talents. In today's economy, this debt would be over $52,800,000 (one talent equals about two hundred pounds of gold). It was an insurmountable liability that the man could not repay. He pleaded for time to pay and the king was merciful, forgiving the entire debt. What a relief that must have been!

Unfortunately, this man then went out and found another who owed him a much smaller debt: a hundred pence, which would be about forty-four dollars. He did not offer this man the same compassion when the man begged for patience. Instead, the unmerciful servant had the man thrown in prison. The king found out about his lack of compassion and dragged the unmerciful man back into his court, asking him the simple question, "Why did you not show him the same mercy as I did to you?"

I realized that God had forgiven my sin just like the king who pardoned the great debt. He expected me to do the same because there is no way that anyone else's debt to me is greater than what I owed Him.

To comprehend forgiving ourselves, we must try to see ourselves as the other person whom the unmerciful servant could not forgive. You must remember that you are not the same person who walked into that abortion clinic. Today you are a different person. You need to forgive your old self just like you'd forgive anyone else involved in your abortion decision.

In Luke 7:36–50, the woman who anointed Jesus was forgiven because she "loved much." The result of her being forgiven is that her faith saved her. We need faith to accept forgiveness, and with that faith comes great love for others. Having the faith to forgive yourself is the same process as forgiving others. It's not tangible nor is it easy, but God can help you.

First John 4:20–21 (NKJV) says, "If someone says, 'I love God,' and hates his brother, he is a liar; for he who does not love his brother whom he has seen, how can he love God whom he has not seen? And this commandment we have from Him [Jesus]: that he who loves God must love his brother also." Later, in 1 John 5:4–5 (NKJV), the author says, "For whatever is born of God overcomes the world. And this is the victory that has overcome the world—our faith. Who is he who overcomes the world, but he who believes that Jesus is the Son of God?"

I understand that this is a tough concept to grasp; I struggled with it myself. You don't like or trust yourself, let alone love yourself. Perhaps "loving yourself" seems prideful, as it did to me. Let's not forget that there is spiritual warfare all around you at this moment, as you are struggling with forgiving and loving yourself. Satan is real and working to keep you from experiencing the love of God. He is the "accuser" as outlined in Revelation 12:10, "for the accuser of our brethren, who accused them before our God day and night, has been cast down." There is more about the devil in Revelation 12:12 (NKJV): "Woe to the inhabitants of the earth and the sea! For the devil has come down to you, having great wrath, because he knows that he has a short time."

Satan thinks he won a great victory in your abortion—one child died and one child (you!) was wounded. He's kept you in bondage for a long time—but Satan often overlooks the power of redemption. Jesus died on the cross for all sin, including abortion. Don't let Satan's lies keep you bound any longer. Ask God to help you break free from those chains. God has redeemed the death of your child by taking your child into His arms, and He longs to do the same with you.

Isaiah 49:15–18 (NKJV) speaks about us, the process of remembering and mourning our children, and God's love for us:

> "Can a woman forget her nursing child, and not have compassion on the son of her womb? Surely they may forget, yet I will not forget you. See, I have inscribed you on the palms of My hands; your walls are continually before Me. Your sons shall make haste; your destroyers and those who laid you waste shall go away from you. Lift up your eyes, look around and see; all these gather together and come to you. As I live," says the Lord, "You shall surely clothe yourselves with them all as an ornament, and bind them on you as a bride does."

He has allowed you to remember and have compassion on your children. He's promised not to forget you. He has your name inscribed on His hands! He will right the wrongs of Satan and bring you to Himself as a bride. It's a beautiful picture of hope and love.

If the concept of forgiving yourself seems impossible, you must remember that nothing is impossible with God. He can help you in this process. Ask Him for help right now and understand that regardless of your emotions or past, God loves you! The pain of a past abortion can be the worst form of self-torture in the world. If you have other children, the very pleasure they bring may deepen your sense of loss. Little League games, piano recitals, Christmas choirs all remind you of what might have been.

If you have no living children, your abortion loss may be even more intense. You may find yourself avoiding parks, schools, and church nurseries in hopes of avoiding the ache of longing they arouse.

Though millions of women share your anguish, only you know the true cost of your abortion. The price has been subtracted from your heart in hundreds of ways, the loss of the child being the most obvious. You may feel tortured with regret over your loss of innocence, over the things you've done in order to cope, over the secrets you've had to keep, and over the physical consequences of the procedure. You likely had your abortion so that your life would not have to change. In reality, the abortion itself forced changes. Changes you never would have chosen.

Even if your life has gone more smoothly than it might have had you not chosen to abort, there is still the fact of the abortion itself. Perhaps you feel secretly guilty for having gone on to attain the things you wanted, when that success has been paid for with your child's life.

Some of us were too young to make this decision and our parents forced the option. The twelve-year-old girl in that room with me awaiting her abortion was likely obeying a parent and may not have had any idea what she was doing. Unless your situation was out of your hands, no matter what pressures you faced, regardless of what misinformation you'd been given, deep down, it could be that the decision was yours. For many women, that truth haunts them like a ghost.

But if God, whose standards are holier than yours, whose hopes for you were even higher than your own—if He has forgiven you, can you not forgive yourself?

Jesus wants so much for you to be free from your sins that He died to make it possible. In John 10:10 (NKJV), He tells us, "I have come that they may have life, and that they may have it more abundantly." You don't need to atone for your abortion by feeling guilty for the rest of your life. The whole point of Christianity is that we could never atone for our sins, whether they are great or small. That's why Jesus came. That's what the cross is all about.

Please, won't you reach out to God and pray? Receive His forgiveness, and begin to forgive yourself. Never assume that your abortion was so great a sin that it cannot be covered by Christ's sacrifice on the cross. God knew that the sins humanity would commit would be great, and He made His sacrifice equally great so that we could live with Him forever in eternity.

Forgiving Others

*I knew I needed to forgive my mother, yet anger toward her con-
sumed me. I asked God to reveal to me ways that I might have hurt her
as well, and He reminded me that I had robbed her of her grandchild,
taking him away from her without even considering her feelings. On
top of that, I had blamed her for his death. As I realized this, my heart
toward her began to change and soften. The understanding that God
forgave me made forgiving her so much easier because I realized she
wasn't responsible for my abortion decision. During the recovery class,
when we began discussing the abortion details, she offered her love to me
by expressing her understanding that she would meet her grandchild in
heaven. She even comforted me with the thought that my two sisters, who
had died in infancy before I was born, were now doting aunts taking care
of their nephew!*

You didn't get pregnant by yourself, and you didn't choose abortion
by yourself. Some of the people involved in your decision know they
were involved—those who counseled you, and naturally, the doctor
who performed the abortion himself. Others may not even know an
abortion took place, but they, too, played a role. Maybe you never
told your parents, your boyfriend, or your friends that you were
pregnant … but you had the abortion so that you never would have
to tell them. In your heart, you still hold them partially responsible.
After all, if they'd been more supportive in other matters, you might
have felt able to go to them with this one.

Maybe you were young and it was your parents' wish, even demand, that you get an abortion. Maybe they took you to the clinic without considering what your wishes might be. You had to obey them.

Yes, the ultimate responsibility is yours. But that doesn't mean it is yours alone. Those who influenced you, wittingly or unwittingly, to make that decision, bear the guilt as well. And though you may be forgiven for your part, you will never be entirely free until you have forgiven them for their part too.

After asking the Lord's help in forgiving Alan for the part he played in my abortion decision, I began to envision him as a twenty-one-year-old boy waiting in the car at the abortion clinic. By speaking to abortion-vulnerable young men, I had learned that many simply looked at abortion as the best answer. They were not considering it as a way to "abuse" their partner. Most men are astounded when I relay the potential of spiritual, emotional, and psychological pain on their loved ones should they choose abortion. I pictured Alan as one of these young men. I remembered the way he hugged me at the bottom of the stairs of the clinic, grateful I was alive. I started to imagine the agony of his emotions while waiting in the car and contemplating that the abortion could take my life. I suddenly realized that he was scared too. In this unplanned pregnancy, his future was at stake as well. I was struck with the truth that had he known what I would endure in that procedure, he may have been supportive of another decision.

Luke 23:34 came to mind, when Jesus prayed before His crucifixion, saying, "Father, forgive them, for they do not know what they are doing."

Alan didn't know what he was doing to me in forcing me into the abortion decision. I needed to offer him the same grace as Jesus did to the crowd. The forgiveness for Alan came in that moment, suddenly, and the anger and betrayal faded away with God's healing touch. Putting myself in this young boy's place helped me know his heart and forgive him the way God asked me to. I never contacted him, but there was a deep release in my heart. What a gift that forgiveness has been in my ministry to young men who are in the same spot!

I understand your pain, but each one of us must come to the point in our journey with the Lord in realizing that forgiveness frees our hearts and releases God's mercy on others.

It's one thing when the person asks to be forgiven. There's something about an apology that makes forgiveness flow more freely. But what about when the person doesn't have any remorse for his or her actions against you? What if the individual does not even comprehend the wrong that he or she has done? Or if the person doesn't even know that he or she was a part of that decision? That's when forgiveness sticks in your throat.

How do we forgive someone who is not sorry—someone who may still think it was the best thing for us or that the abortion was no big deal? First, it is important to look at what forgiveness is not. It is not:

- **excusing** them for their actions
- **forgetting** what they did to us
- **understanding** why they did what they did
- **trusting** them again, because trust must be earned.

Forgiving without repentance feels like acceptance of the wrong done. It feels as if you are saying, "That's okay," when it isn't okay. When it was a big deal.

God never asks us to approve what was done, to condone the wrong. He just wants us to stop holding them accountable for it— and let Him hold them accountable instead. As we're reminded in Romans 14:10, "we will all stand before God's judgment seat."

The commands in Scripture to forgive others are numerous:

- "If you hold anything against anyone, forgive him" (Mark 11:25).
- "Be reconciled to your brother" (Matt. 5:24).
- "I tell you ... seventy-seven times" (Matt. 18:22).

The list goes on and on.

It often feels like a tall order. But God never asks us to do anything that is not, ultimately, good for us. Our unforgiveness doesn't affect them, but us! It's like a fatal venom that destroys our peace and is harmless toward the offenders.

Do you know how the dictionary defines the word *forgive*? "To renounce anger or resentment against an offender."[1] Wouldn't that be nice? Imagine it. To cease to feel resentment ... to cease to feel resentment ... When was the last time you experienced that, the absence of resentment? Do you even remember what it was like?

Your heavenly Father would like you to be experiencing that now. He's not asking you to say it didn't matter. It did matter. If you were lied to, misinformed, it mattered. If you were pressured or

threatened, it mattered. If you felt alone, afraid, in danger of rejection, it mattered. If you were made to feel responsible for someone
else's emotional well-being, it mattered. It mattered to God then, and
it matters to Him now. His forgiveness is available to those people,
but that is between them and Him. What He asks is that you put the
burden of resentment in His hands. Forgive them. Let them off the
hook in your heart, and allow God to put them on His hook, to deal
with in His own way.

As you do so, ask Him to show you a new way to view those
people, new insights into who they are and why. And too, ask Him
to show you what responsibility you might have in the tensions that
did, or perhaps still do, exist in those relationships. He'd like few
things more than to clear the slate between you and those people—
to replace resentment with understanding and reconciliation.

Make a list of everyone who had a part, big or small, known
or unknown, in your abortion decision. Explore thoroughly your
reasons for resenting them. Then pray through your list, asking God
to help you see them in a new light, to forgive them, and to turn
them over to Him for repayment of their debt.

*Recently, I faced my birth father and my stepmother, the woman
my father had left us to be with. I had rarely been in her presence and
had never honestly expressed any emotions concerning her role in the
destruction of my family. In a quiet and gentle discussion about the
past, her voice rose in pain as she said, "I want you to know that you've
hurt me and caused me a great deal of heartache!" If God had not*

already healed the anger I felt toward this woman, my response would have been much different and possibly destructive.

But in that moment of truth, the Lord's power came over my heart. I realized that I owed her an apology. Because of the depth of pain she'd caused in my family, I had justified my negative actions toward her and never considered that I may have hurt her deeply as well. God's power assisted me in calmly and openly acknowledging the sins I had committed and asking for her forgiveness. The reaction of my love and repentance silenced the angry emotion in the room. While she refrained from providing direct confirmation of her forgiveness toward me, I was released at a deep level and filled with joy. I later thanked the Lord for the opportunity to ask for her forgiveness and, in doing so, was able to completely forgive her as well.

No Contact

Please understand that forgiving someone does not mean you should contact him or her. It is not a good thing to relay that you forgive people when they don't believe they are guilty of any wrongdoing. Points like "You were wrong but I forgive you" are not a productive way of forgiving but only serve to shame the other person into an apology. True forgiveness doesn't require an apology but resides in our hearts before the Lord.

I strongly discourage post-abortive women from contacting the fathers of their aborted children, especially during the healing process, unless this person is their spouse. When we go through deep recollection periods, often we feel drawn to these individuals from our past. If you are married or in a relationship—or if the father of your child is in a similar situation—contact is not recommended, even if you have good motives and no intention of entering into a relationship with the person. These memories are best brought to the Lord, confessed, and left in His hands. Paul's words in 1 Thessalonians 4:3–5, 7 outline this perfectly; "It is God's will that you should be sanctified: that you should avoid sexual immorality; that each of you should learn to control his own body in a way that is holy and honorable, not in passionate lust like the heathen, who do not know God.... For God did not call us to be impure, but to live a holy life."

....

Blessed is he
whose transgressions are forgiven,
whose sins are covered.
Blessed is the man
whose sin the LORD does not count against him
and in whose spirit is no deceit.
When I kept silent,
my bones wasted away
through my groaning all day long.
For day and night
your hand was heavy upon me;
my strength was sapped
as in the heat of summer.
Then I acknowledged my sin to you
and did not cover up my iniquity.
I said, "I will confess

my transgressions to the LORD"—
and you forgave
the guilt of my sin.
Therefore let everyone who is godly pray to you
while you may be found;
surely when the mighty waters rise,
they will not reach him.
You are my hiding place;
you will protect me from trouble
and surround me with songs of deliverance.

—Psalm 32:1–7

....

Get rid of all bitterness, rage and anger, brawling
and slander,
along with every form of malice.
Be kind and compassionate to one another, forgiving
each other,
just as in Christ God forgave you.

—Ephesians 4:31–32

....

Chapter 6

Sharing the Secret of Abortion

For there is nothing hidden that will not be
disclosed, and nothing concealed that will not
be known or brought out into the open.
—*Luke 8:17*

If you are like most post-abortive women, there are significant people in your life who do not know that you have had an abortion. You may have good reasons for your silence. But then again, the reason may be pure and simple fear. Do you find that this secret is eroding some of your relationships? Does it stand between you and true intimacy with someone in your life? Perhaps it is time to take this particular scrapbook off the shelf and open it up. The time may or may not be right to share, but it is certainly something to prayerfully consider, especially with regard to your immediate family.

Perhaps the greatest element preventing post-abortive women from sharing the secret of our abortion is the fear that our confessions will lead to judgment and rejection. Our unhealed hearts often sit in silent prisons of pain longing for spiritual, emotional, and even physical release. The key to our prison doors can often lie in hearing someone else talk about abortion, speaking directly to us with compassion.

To the confessor, sharing can be liberating because a great deal of energy is expended in maintaining this secret. Jesus was clear that the power of truth is freeing in John 8:31–32: "If you hold to my teaching, you are really my disciples. Then you will know the truth, and the truth will set you free." Whether the confession is publicly or privately revealed, it is powerful in breaking Satan's grip of shame on wounded hearts.

A Biblical Example—Esther

Esther is perhaps the best biblical example of a woman who was used by God to speak. It's good for all of us to go back and read the story of Esther. God knew the story's end before Esther was born. He had a plan set when Nebuchadnezzar took Mordecai into captivity. God made Esther beautiful so the king would easily fall in love with her. While she was placed in great danger and could have been killed for her actions, God protected her and kept her safe from all harm. God also dealt justice to those who were against His people.

Esther didn't embrace Mordecai's request for her to go to the king uninvited but argued that obedience could result in her death. He then reminded her that perhaps God made her queen for this reason (Est. 4:1–14). That point made her embrace the task of speaking to her husband in order to save the lives of her people. Esther was a woman who did not question God (as far as we know). She trusted Him and was prepared to perish in order to obey Him (Est. 4:16).

Esther was patient and prepared in great detail for God's assign-
ment with the king. She worked hard to earn his respect and admiration
by being humble in front of him. When her unrequested presence was
sanctioned by the king, she simply invited him to dinner. When he
came, he offered her half his kingdom. Esther didn't respond except to
invite him to another dinner. Between the two meals, God gave Esther
some encouragement when He reminded the king that Mordecai had
saved his life and he had done nothing to reward him. I'm sure the
added confidence of Mordecai being honored at Haman's expense
helped Esther at the next dinner. The rest, as they say, is history....

Esther was used by God to deliver an entire nation. She argued
at first because the task could have cost her life. Once she accepted
the task, she prepared herself with prayer and fasting. God's hand
certainly was upon her heart and He went ahead and paved the way
so that she would be protected. The result was unexpected elevation
of her family and people.

The Power of Our Testimonies

My first question on that initial night of my post-abortion-recovery
class was, "Are you going to make us tell anyone?" I was relieved to
discover that encouraging public confession wasn't the purpose of
the class. After experiencing God's healing, His call would come to
my life to share publicly. This led to a great struggle within my heart,
but God eventually brought me to full surrender. Each time I share,
I relive the horror of my abortion, visualizing my child's death, and
then reexperience God's healing touch.

God is not a God of secrets. Jesus spoke in Matthew 6:4–18
about only three things that we should keep secret: fasting, giving,

and prayer. Revelation 12:11 outlines the power of the testimony over Satan's work: "They overcame him [Satan] by the blood of the Lamb, and by the word of their testimony."

Secrets can bind us to sin. Family and friends need to hear the truth from the loved one before it is relayed through third-party channels. One woman told me that her ex-husband had casually told their teenage daughter about their abortion years earlier. It appeared that the father's motive was to belittle the woman in the eyes of her daughter during a custody battle. He neglected to share his own role in coercing her abortion decision. The daughter was very angry with her mother. God moved and allowed a peaceful discussion between mother and daughter that led to a stronger bond of love and understanding. That mother relayed that she should have been honest in the first place because the truth would have been much easier from her lips.

In 1991, when the Lord spoke to my heart and asked me to first share my abortion testimony to a small gathering of staff at Focus on the Family, I reacted like Jonah. I said "No!" God was patient and gave me several weeks to prepare. While He would confirm this calling many times, I actively fled from even considering the idea. His calling became louder and I fought harder. God's hand was heavy upon me and finally, on the morning of the scheduled devotions, I hung my head and agreed to obey Him. As always with God, the results of my obedience were incredible. There wasn't a greater group of individuals to hear my first confession. They received me with love and honor and still pray for me today.

A few days later a Focus on the Family broadcast producer called to ask if I had a testimony of someone who had an abortion. Quickly I replied, "Well, you can always use mine!" As soon as I said those words, I froze in fear. I didn't have any time to think about my offer because in less than an hour I was recording my testimony for Dr. Dobson. It was the first time in my life that I can remember what it felt like to be God's vessel. I don't remember a word because God did all the talking! Dr. Dobson wrote me an encouraging note about my testimony, relaying that it would be featured on an upcoming broadcast.

That reality hit me like a brick because it meant ten million listeners would know about my abortion. They offered me the option to share anonymously but I said, "No. Please share my name. God wants me to be visible so that I can help others." Again, I didn't know where the words came from, because I wanted to take them back right away! God was directing my words and I knew I must obey.

While Tom and a few others knew this truth, I needed to share this secret with family and friends before they heard my very public testimony. I couldn't take the risk of someone hearing about my abortion via a public broadcast. I made a list of the individuals and wrote each a letter and sent a copy of my testimony tape. Incredibly, out of twenty-five letters, only two people responded. A benefit of this process was that God made it clear who were my "true" friends. Later He would replace each lost friend with many more!

Two days before the broadcast I was in a panic over the fact that I was actually sharing my story with millions. I was scared, frightened, and overwhelmed at the potential for rejection. I tried to accept that I couldn't remove my name from the tape since it had already been distributed to stations. God stepped in at that point to provide yet another confirmation and put my heart to rest.

I was put on hold during a business call and an old familiar Keith Green song, "Asleep in the Light," was playing (www.KeithGreen.com). I had loved this song before the abortion but hadn't heard it in years. God gave me a very clear and poignant message through the following words:

You see the need; you hear the cries, so how can you delay?

God's calling, and you're the one, but like Jonah you run,

He's told you to speak but you keep holding it in.

Oh can't you see it's such sin.[1]

With all my heart, I knew that God had used the song to give me a strong message about the impact of my sacrifice in sharing publicly. Millions could be reached with the hope of His healing.

Sharing with Spouses

One of the first questions many post-abortive women ask themselves is *Should I tell my husband?* I believe that the answer is yes. When I met my husband, my heart reasoned that if he was going to reject me because of this choice it would be better to know that before my heart was too invested. So I shared this truth with him shortly after we began seeing each other. My sharing the truth was like Ruth lying at Boaz's feet, hoping that he'd accept her as his wife and not reject her (Ruth 3). For many women, laying out this truth openly to present or future spouses requires a strong act of courage and faith in God.

The room was dark when I told Tom about my abortion. He held me close and comforted me as I cried. He told me that if I had been pregnant with his baby I never would have found my way to an abortion clinic. He also made a surprising confession: He understood my pain because his former girlfriend had aborted his unborn child behind his back. I had never thought that men could share the same grief over their aborted children. The truth helped me understand his heart and trust him at a far deeper level. I fell in love with him even more after that moment.

In his song, *Honesty*, Billy Joel laments that "Honesty is such a lonely word, everyone is so untrue. Honesty is hardly ever heard, but mostly what I need from you." This secular song portrays what most of us want in a relationship—to be able to trust the other person with every part of our hearts.

Many women are hesitant to share with their husbands because this secret impacts the element of trust. There is always a possibility that the spouse will be more upset about her withholding the secret than the fact the wife had chosen abortion in the past.

Many women are hampered by the belief that sharing this truth with their spouses could end their marriage, which could damage present children. What a relief it is when they discover after summoning the courage that the marriage can not only survive this truth but also can flourish at a new level of intimacy due to the understanding that their husbands love them *in spite of* this secret. Many husbands express relief because they felt there was a secret lurking in their marriage and appreciate their wives' honesty in trusting them with the truth.

Once, I was sitting next to a particularly chatty man on an airplane. When he came to that common question, "What do you do for a living?" I told him that I worked with pregnancy care centers. The passenger remarked that his church supported a local pregnancy center, and he was intrigued as to the focus of my educational efforts.

When I shared that I had personally experienced abortion and educated specifically on reaching post-abortive hearts, his face froze.

Quietly, he told me that his wife had experienced abortion twice in her past. He said, "She told me about it when we first started going out and I wasn't judgmental. But we never talked about it again. It seems like a taboo topic and that bothers me." He expressed he didn't want to cause her more pain by bringing up such an emotional subject, but he was concerned that her lack of obvious regret about this topic indicated a potential "cold" heart.

This man listened intently as I shared about post-abortion syndrome and how we work hard to forget this truth. I encouraged him not to think the worst about his wife's inability to open herself up to the pain that may be lurking in her heart. Then I suggested he broach the topic with his wife in a compassionate manner, offering her this book and sharing that he doesn't judge her but wants to know more about this part of her past. I have had many such divine appointments with men who want to openly speak about this past choice in their wives' lives but are afraid to cause more pain.

As long as you are not in an abusive relationship, I believe your present or future spouse deserves to know the truth about your past choices. This can be the first step in building a stronger marriage.

Sharing with Children

Many post-abortive individuals are exceptionally fearful of sharing this secret with their children. This fear is based on two elements—that their children could think less of them or that this truth could encourage sexual activity outside of marriage. Being bound to secrets is a troubling thing, especially when our children could repeat our same mistakes!

There are also times when the couple has shared the decision to abort, and are still together. There needs to be full agreement between the spouses in order to share with children. If there isn't a mutual accord, respect should be shown and sharing the truth delayed. God must lead each individual in the details of sharing this secret. If you experienced abortion before you met your current spouse, I believe your husband should still provide his approval prior to any discussion with his children.

My oldest son was seven when the topic of abortion came up. Since I was working full time in the pregnancy care ministry, abortion was a common word in our home. "Mommy, what's abortion?" Bruce asked. I took a deep breath and replied, "Abortion is when they take a baby out of his mother's belly before it is big enough to survive. The baby goes to live with Jesus and the mommy can be very sad." Bruce instantly realized the horror I was describing. His eyes grew large as he asked, "Is that legal, Mommy?" My response was, "Yes, honey, it's legal. My job is to help mommies who are thinking about this choice because many do not know they are carrying a fully formed baby."

I allowed Bruce a few months to absorb the abortion issue. From time to time he'd ask other questions, always overwhelmed that it was a legal option. I waited a few months before sharing with him the secret of my own abortion. When God opened the door, I didn't share many details, but Bruce wasn't horrified nor did he think less of me. When I asked him to forgive me for allowing them to take his big brother, he hugged me and gracefully gave it. Over the following days he asked questions but was never judgmental. Some years later, we were talking about regrets and he said, "I know your biggest regret, Mom. Losing my older brother." He went on to say, "If he were alive, I probably wouldn't be here, right, Mom?" I was searching to determine if he felt any "survival guilt" in this question and responded, "Yes, that could be, but that wasn't God's plan. In spite of my bad choice, He gave me you as a son. He planned all the days of your life and has a great purpose for you." Bruce was blessed with that confirmation!

Several years later I shared in the same manner with my second son, Michael. I again started by telling him about abortion itself. He looked at me with his big blue eyes and said, "Oh, Mommy, I'm so glad you didn't abort me." I hugged him and waited a while before sharing about his brother. When the Lord told me the time was right to share the truth, I took Michael on a "date" to the mall. I brought up the *abortion* word again and shared quietly that I had been one of those girls who made that choice. I told him about his big brother. He responded excitedly, "I have a big brother in heaven?" "Yes, you do, Michael. Do you forgive me for allowing him to die?" He turned to me and hugged me. He said, "Yes, Mom, I forgive you." Then he went on dreaming about his brother.

When Michael was thirteen, he overheard a news report where someone was promoting abortion rights. He got very angry and said, "I think anyone who has an abortion should go to jail for life!" I was quite shocked at his reaction, but understood the outrage. I asked quietly, "Do you think I should be in jail too, Michael?" My dear boy looked at me and said, "Yes, sometimes I do." Thankfully my healed heart was prepared for his reaction. God gave me the words to voice, "You know, sometimes I feel that way too, Michael. But abortion isn't considered homicide in our nation and God has given me a role to help other women making that choice."

That didn't settle the matter between us; I knew that Michael simply didn't understand why women choose abortion. A few weeks later I took him along with me on a speaking engagement where he sat with his bright blue eyes watching me intently while I talked about my abortion experience. The Lord's blessing flowed into his youthful mind and when I left the podium, my son embraced me, kissed me on the cheek, and whispered into my ear, "That was wonderful, Mom." Never again would he judge a woman for an abortion choice, because he understood that we didn't approach our choice in a murderous mind-set.

When it comes to an abstinence perspective, our children truly need to understand that sexual activity outside of marriage can result in unplanned pregnancy situations where abortions may be considered. My oldest was dating a girl in high school whose parents were adamantly pro-choice. When Bruce drove to visit them, his "choose-life" license plates spoke volumes. He said that her father mentioned the plates and Bruce was not hesitant to share his own thoughts on the issue. The two "agreed to disagree" at that point.

After he told me about this encounter, I spoke to him about what could happen should his girlfriend become pregnant. Bruce was indignant and said, "I'd never encourage her to have an abortion, Mother." I said, "It may not be up to you, Bruce. The baby's father has no rights in an abortion decision. Her parents believe in abortion and have big dreams for her life. If she came up pregnant, they may insist on an abortion." His eyes grew wide as he realized the truth of my point. He said, "Then she would be wounded for life, and so would I. And you and Dad as well." Immediately a unique abstinence perspective was entrenched in his memory. He did not lose his virginity in that relationship.

If there is someone in your life whom you are afraid to tell about your abortion, start in prayer. Sharing about an abortion can open a lot of doors to healing in a relationship. It can also prevent the same sin from occurring in future generations and prevent abortion from being considered in future unplanned pregnancy situations. How sad it is when the post-abortive individual becomes a post-abortive grandparent. If the Lord is leading you to share this secret, ask God to provide confirmation as to the perfect time to share. Be ready when the door opens and understand that God has gone before you to prepare your loved ones' hearts with the truth.

Sharing with Extended Family

A woman once wrote to me after reading my story and shared a lovely story about her relationship with her mother. Her mother never knew the truth of her abortion and was now dying of cancer. Monica wanted to talk to her about it, but it was too late—her mother could no longer communicate. As she sat by her mother's bedside one day, pondering this fact and looking through this book, her mother kept repeating a number. After a while, Monica turned to that page number in the book and found there a special verse that gave her comfort about that situation. God used her mother to reach her heart that day.

In my own family relations, sharing the truth has involved losing friendships. My pregnant relative Elisa was stunned when I told her I was attending a post-abortion-recovery class. She said that before she had met her husband, she had chosen abortion, and that her parents wanted her to abort the child she was now carrying because they didn't think her husband would support her financially.

All through her response, I sensed deep pain, denial, and justification of her abortion. My story had opened up a wound in her heart that was barely covered. She ended by saying, "While I'm glad I didn't abort this baby, the other was conceived in a one-night stand and I still believe that was the best decision." Our relationship changed after that. Elisa didn't wait for my response but collected herself and left the room. She was never alone with me again.

My heart went out to her. The consequences of my quick confession meant that every time she saw me she was reminded of her abortion. There was nothing I could do to change that fact. She didn't know the Lord and was simply trying to get through her pregnancy, which was already a huge reminder of her loss. While I wanted to help her heal, I couldn't. All I could do is pray for her. I believe the Lord ordained the conversation because at least Elisa knew that her eventual emotional pain could be related to her abortion. In His time, I believe the Lord will bring other people into her life to help her heal.

There are some situations where sharing this truth may not be in the Lord's plan. Prayer is the only way to determine this. Many times, the elderly cannot handle the burden of this truth. Like the woman who asked me to forgive her for having an affair with my father, truth can provide an undue burden on hearts that were not intended to bear the weight of this truth. While this may prohibit you from sharing your abortion secret publicly, it can be that the Lord is closing the door to prepare your heart at another level.

Sharing with Those Considering Abortion

There is nothing that delights my heart more than to allow God to use me in speaking directly to men and women who are considering abortion. Each week these individuals call or e-mail Ramah International. Quietly they ask if I can refer them to an abortion clinic. I normally respond, "What is your situation?" In the ensuing moments I hear various angles of the same story—abortion seems like the best option.

Men and women often leap to the abortion option without even confirming they are pregnant! My goal with each call is to listen to their perspectives, quietly relay that I have chosen abortion and ask them what they know about this option. Through listening I've realized that after all these years, abortion still is an unknown procedure. Most will admit they fear "regretting" the choice but see no alternatives. Each time I share my abortion story the listener responds positively, thanking me for being so honest. While I may never know the decision they make, I always let them know that even if they choose abortion, I'll be here to help.

What a joy it is to provide them with information about their local pregnancy care center that can verify their pregnancy, possibly introduce them to their unborn child through an ultrasound screen, and equip them with information about abortion's risks at psychological, spiritual, emotional, and physical levels. Many appreciate just having a calm voice on the line that understands their situation and wants to help. Many of us are not called to share publicly. Privately shared, our stories can make a life-changing difference. At the end of this book is more information on how each of us can participate in positive life efforts to end abortion one life at a time.

Sharing at a Public Level

Aborted Women: Silent No More by David Reardon was one of the first books I read when I entered the positive-life arena. The stories it contained allowed me to understand that my pain was typical and that many of my apprehensions in life could be related to my past abortion choice. God made it obvious to my heart a few weeks later that my calling involved sharing my struggle through abortion and the redemption Christ gave me in order to help other women find the same hope in God's healing.

As I have matured, I've watched how some well-meaning individuals encourage and solicit the post-abortive testimony for various "awareness" efforts against legalized abortion. Sharing publicly is actually a rare calling because of the intense responsibility and spiritual maturity that is required.

Public testifiers must be trained, equipped, and accomplished in the healing process before even contemplating this mission. This leadership position is outlined in 1 Timothy 3:1–7:

> If anyone sets his heart on being an overseer, he desires a noble task. Now the overseer must be above reproach … temperate, self-controlled, respectable, hospitable, able to teach, not given to drunkenness, not violent but gentle, not quarrelsome, not a lover of money.… He must not be a recent convert, or he may become conceited and fall under the same judgment as the devil. He must also have a good reputation with outsiders, so that he will not fall into disgrace and into the devil's trap.

Being "silent no more" at a public level requires a great deal of spiritual maturity. Each testimony should begin with a prayer, asking God to use us as His vessel, taking comfort in the words of 2 Peter

1:21: "prophecy never had its origins in the will of man, but men spoke from God as they were carried along by the Holy Spirit."

For those of you who feel called to speak publicly, you must first be "silent no more" with friends and family. It is important that they hear your truth from your heart first versus from someone else.

Before you speak publicly, here are a few questions you should prayerfully contemplate:

- Is it God who is calling you to speak?
- Are you seeking attention or reward?
- Have you shared this story with family and friends first?
- Do you think that sharing can cleanse you of sin?
- Do your spouse and children support your sharing?
- Will you focus your message on God?
- Are you trained to assist those who may respond?

After a few years at Focus on the Family, when I was traveling and speaking extensively, my boss and mentor, H. B. London Jr., took me aside. He said, "Sydna, I want to warn you about the potential for a spirit of pride to overcome you in this work. You must fight that possibility, always giving the praise and glory to God. The more humble you are, the more God can speak through you." Every time I speak, I experience humiliation and pain in the confession of my abortion. The only joy is in sharing how the Lord healed my heart. If I ever get to the point when this testimony doesn't hurt, I'll know it's time to quit. After all these years, I know what H. B. was saying—it's only worth it if God gets all the glory.

Repairing a Poorly Shared Secret

After an abortion, it's possible that you may have hurt people with this truth. Many post-abortive women defend their actions venomously, even to family and friends in an effort to justify their abortion decisions. The anger emotion pushes many in this behavior and it can easily hurt others. God may be calling you to apologize for past behavior that occurred through your wounding and denial in poorly sharing this secret.

About a year after my abortion, I was riding the wave of relief and denial, smoking pot each day and justifying my decision to myself. I moved to a secular state college and established myself specifically with pro-abortion friends. My abortion had ended my crisis, and I firmly believed abortion had been the best choice in my circumstances. Over dinner with my brother and his wife, I casually interjected my abortion into the conversation, saying, "That was around the time I had my abortion...." My brother responded, "You had a what?" I said, "Oh, an abortion. Didn't you know about that? I thought you did." They both became upset and the dinner ended abruptly. It was the first negative reaction I had ever received, and I grew angry with them. I never realized the sword this secret could have been to their hearts and that their negative response could have been more accurately described as horror and grief.

Ten years later, during my healing classes, I was reminded of this specific memory and was convicted that I had hurt them with this truth. The next time I saw them, I apologized for my behavior during that incident,

but the topic spurred a bad memory in their hearts. My sister-in-law com-
mented, "We would have adopted your child, Sydna." I gently reminded
her that she hadn't even been in my brother's life during the time of the
abortion, so adoption could never have been an option. She quietly changed
the subject. While I am still unsure that forgiveness has been granted, I am
at peace with the Lord in addressing this sin from my past.

We must be careful about how we share about this fact of our
past with loved ones. God will remind you of people in your past
that you could have hurt with this truth as well. I realize that my
brother lost a nephew in the abortion. My sister-in-law couldn't
walk in my shoes and understand my wounding in making this
choice. My ongoing dysfunctional behavior around that period,
which included smoking pot in front of them, only reinforced
their perspective that I was a true prodigal, perhaps unworthy of
redemption.

Out of the blue, I received a call from Alan's father, a pastor. I had
sent him a broadcast tape of my story two years earlier but had never
heard from him. He relayed to me then that he and his wife rarely talked
about this loss and that she couldn't speak to me over the phone. They
were still grieving. He said that Alan had just married a woman with
two older children and so had probably aborted his only child. He fin-
ished the conversation by saying that they had forgiven me and were very
proud of my efforts.

While the Lord forgives us our sins, that doesn't automatically mean others can. If you aborted a child of a man who wanted the child, you know the anger and rejection you may have received in breaking his heart. The letter I wrote to Alan's father to confess about my abortion before the Focus on the Family broadcast went unanswered for two years, but all the while the Lord was moving in his heart, reminding him of my name and the need for forgiveness. When he finally called me, offering his support, he also had a request—that I not reveal Alan's family's name publicly as they had not shared the secret with others. It was too much for him to bear to speak about the abortion as I did. In return for his wonderful encouragement and love, protecting his identity was a simple request.

Luke 7:36–50 (NKJV) is a beautiful passage that speaks about the amazing love that comes when someone has been "forgiven much." Jesus was at the home of Simon the Pharisee when a woman "who was a sinner" came and began to wash His feet with her tears and dried them with her hair. Jesus noticed the look of disdain on the Pharisee's face. He told him the parable about two people who were forgiven debts. One man owed more money than the other. He asked the judgmental man, "Tell Me, therefore, which of them will love him more?" Simon said, "I suppose the one whom he forgave more." The point Jesus wanted to make is in verse 47: "Therefore I say to you, her sins, which are many, are forgiven, for she loved much. But to whom little is forgiven, the same loves little."

If you need to repent to someone in your life who was wounded by this choice, pray for the opportunity to offer this apology. Ask the Lord to confirm this leading and prepare their hearts to discuss this loss in their lives. Keep in mind that their forgiving you isn't the

point of the exercise. Offering your humble confession is the step
that Christ requires when we have offended or hurt others. In the
end, He may need to work on their hearts in helping them offer you
the same compassion in return.

....

Do not cast me from your presence,
or take your Holy Spirit from me.
Restore to me the joy of your salvation
and grant me a willing spirit, to sustain me.
Then I will teach transgressors your ways,
and sinners will turn back to you.
Save me from bloodguilt, O God,
the God who saves me,
and my tongue will sing of your righteousness.
O Lord, open my lips,
and my mouth will declare your praise.

—Psalm 51:11–15

....

Chapter 7

A River of Tears: Grieving Your Loss

The hearts of the people cry out to the Lord.
O wall of the Daughter of Zion,
let your tears flow like a river day and night;
give yourself no relief, your eyes no rest.
Arise, cry out in the night, as the
watches of the night begin;
pour out your heart like water in
the presence of the Lord.
Lift up your hands to him for the
lives of your children.
—Lamentations 2:18–19

I remember being alone in my dorm room seven months after the abortion ... near the time that I should have been giving birth. I refused to think about my abortion, but my body's time clock was signaling the truth. A friend—not even a close friend—had betrayed me that week. I found myself crying as though I'd never stop. All night long I cried, until my eyes were swollen shut. I even considered suicide, and I made up my mind never to trust anyone again. It was obviously an overreaction, but it would be years before I could acknowledge the true source of my pain that night. I was subconsciously grieving the death of my unborn child during the week he would have been born.

It is terrifying for many to consider actually mourning the loss of their aborted children. Tears of remorse are difficult to release because we fear that these emotions will consume us. The looming presence of this pain may drive us to great fear. Thoughts of suicide may creep in and out of our minds because it sounds easier than touching that pain. Often we ignore it or deny it.

But God has not forgotten us. We are as visible to Him now as we were before the abortion. He will be there to help us clear away the rubble that is left from our walls. What we fear is the pain of the truth, our guilt and shame. We don't want to hurt anymore. What He knows is that the darkness of these secrets can shield us from the light of His mercy and grace.

Regardless of your current emotions about the legality of abortion, the first step in healing normally comes when you acknowledge your baby as a lost child and allow yourself to begin to grieve his or her loss. If you were to lose a baby after a live birth, or if you were to miscarry a child you wanted, you would expect to grieve, and deeply.

And in the process of mourning, you would begin to heal. There is no denying that a life is extinguished in each abortion.

The thought of grieving a baby that you chose to abort in the first place seems so contrary. You may have been told that since it wasn't really a baby to begin with, there is nothing to grieve—so you have resisted those feelings.

Yet even though this baby was lost by choice, you have nevertheless lost a child. Your heart still needs to grieve. It is that grief that will break down the wall. You needn't be afraid of the pain. God will walk through it with you. Though you may cry for days yet to come, remember:

> Those who sow in tears
> > will reap with songs of joy.
> He who goes out weeping,
> > carrying seed to sow,
> will return with songs of joy,
> > carrying sheaves with him. (Ps. 126:5–6)

Remember when David committed adultery with Bathsheba, then had Uriah killed? When the child died, David comforted Bathsheba, who was grieving. And when Lazarus died and was in the tomb, Jesus, even knowing full well that He was about to restore life, showed us how to mourn the loss of someone we love. The Bible very simply says, "Jesus wept" (John 11:35). It is okay to cry, to weep great tears of sorrow over the loss of a loved one. That is how we can release the pent-up grief, how we can mourn our loss and begin to grow stronger in the Lord.

God developed the concept of mourning to allow us a way to release the pain of loss. It is a human trait to need closure after the death of a loved one. Funerals and wakes are all "passage" rituals that ensure mourning and encourage tears.

Sometimes the process is quick. But usually, the destruction of the wall around our hearts takes months or even years. Maybe the pain is too great to deal with all at once, or maybe we resist the process. You may take down a load of bricks only to mortar half of them back in place again. But be patient. Enjoy the rays of light that will sometimes stream through the cracks. And when the grief threatens to overwhelm you, look forward to the days that are promised in Isaiah 60:20 (NKJV): "For the LORD will be your everlasting light, and the days of your mourning shall be ended."

What an incredible promise! How wonderful to know that your days of sorrow will end! The thing that you've been so afraid of will be behind you forever. Never again will you live in darkness or fear. The wall will no longer be necessary, because God's love has released you from your sin.

I remember the orientation program on my first day at Focus on the Family. I was apprehensive of the Christian environment, concerned that if they discovered that I had chosen abortion, I could be fired. Then they showed Dr. James Dobson, founder of that ministry, on a video sharing about his views on abortion. I'll never forget the moment when he said, "I know I am speaking to many women who have chosen abortion. I want you to know that there is no sin that God can't forgive. The problem

*may be you don't forgive yourself and you may need help in that area."
Suddenly, a wall within my heart was broken down. I felt safe for the
first time in many years. I was working in an organization that clearly
wouldn't judge me. The next day I discovered a Focus on the Family
booklet titled "Identifying and Overcoming Post-Abortion Syndrome."
With shaking hands, I opened the resource.*

*There it was in black and white. The booklet described the classic
symptoms of post-abortion syndrome (described on pages 50–55) and I
had many of them evident in my life. Now I knew why the third week of
March was always hard—it was the anniversary of my baby's due date.
It took all my courage, but I dialed the number of the pregnancy care
center and enrolled in their post-abortion-recovery class. And the walls
began to come down.*

It's important to remember that God is no stranger to pain. His
people experienced pain throughout the Old Testament. The psalms,
as well as the book of Job, are filled with tears. Lamentations (which
means "funeral songs") was most likely written by the prophet Jeremiah, grieving about the destruction of Jerusalem.

If the Lord created us in His own image, He created our tears as
well, and He wants to use them to make us stronger. In being able
to cry, you bring yourself humbly before the Lord. Pride is dissolved
and the love you have stored in your heart is released. Tears indicate
love for the child you lost so many years ago.

The First Step Toward Peace

Tears can be the first step toward peace in your heart over your abortion experience. Again I am reminded of the passage in Luke 7 when

Jesus was anointed by a sinful woman. While the passage doesn't reveal her name, it states that she had lived a sinful life. Verse 38 (NKJV) shares the story of how her tears endeared her to Jesus: "and stood at His feet behind Him weeping; and she began to wash His feet with her tears, and wiped them with the hair of her head; and she kissed His feet and anointed them with the fragrant oil."

Jesus' reaction to her tears was love and admiration. He informed the judgmental Pharisee in verse 47 that "her many sins have been forgiven—for she loved much." Later He spoke to her directly and said, "Your faith has saved you; go in peace."

Realize that your tears are precious and God wants to use them to ease your pain and increase your faith. This release means that the walls are coming down and His love can flow freely into your heart. Open up and give yourself permission to cry.

A Time to Mourn

The Bible is very clear that there are to be set times of mourning. For example, read Ecclesiastes 3:1 and 4:

> There is a time for everything ...
> a time to weep and a time to laugh,
>   a time to mourn and a time to dance.

In biblical times, people wore sackcloth and ashes to inform the world of their emotions. While our society believes that you should swallow the pain and "get over it," God didn't make us that way. He designed our grieving times to be events that bring us closer to Him for comfort. Consider the words of Psalm 23:4: "Even though I walk through the valley of the shadow of death, I will fear no evil, for you are with me; your rod and your staff, they comfort me."

It is not uncommon for women going through post-abortion grief to cry for long periods of time. It is also possible that the woman cannot cry. Sometimes we cry because of triggers—a song on the radio that reminds us of the abortion period in our life, seeing the father of our aborted child, meeting a child the same age our child would have been. While you may feel as though you are going crazy because you cannot predict your tears, realize that your reaction is normal.

When emotions have been bottled up inside for so many years, they can overcome us like an ocean wave hitting the beach. We don't know which way is up and we can't find a solid footing. But just as soon as the wave of emotions launches upon our hearts, it rolls back into the ocean leaving us feeling out of breath and trying to stabilize ourselves before the next wave hits.

The main thing to remember about grief is that you don't get over it—you get through it. Grief doesn't touch everyone the same way. Many women going through abortion-recovery classes in local pregnancy care centers or churches watch others cry openly, yet remain completely calm and rational themselves. They have kept these emotions at bay for so many years that it takes exposure to the truth to break down their wall of composure. Maybe it isn't until a point of discussion blasts open a hole in their emotional wall that their true feelings finally hit them. At this point, tears pour out for days on end. Then, all of a sudden, they are finished crying. Never judge another person's grieving methods. God made us all unique individuals for His own purposes.

Getting Through the Pain

You might be asking yourself, *How long am I going to feel this pain? Will I ever be normal again?* You will never be the same person you were before the abortion, but you can experience peace and healing in time. Give yourself permission to take as long as you need to grieve. If you need to walk slowly, painfully, deliberately through the center of your grief, go right ahead. But while you can lean on others, the work of getting through grief lies squarely on your own shoulders. Keep in mind that you are experiencing a normal reaction to death, no matter how long ago your child died. When you have chosen abortion multiple times, your grief can be understandably intensified.

Each person must discover the coping skills that work best for her. Sometimes talking with a close and trustworthy friend, minister, or counselor, sharing your feelings about your lost child is comforting. Pets can also be therapeutic because they are nonjudgmental companions whose only role is to love us. Many individuals find solace in reading psalms or books about how other people deal with grief.

As I mentioned earlier, journaling is an excellent way to release emotions and bring you to greater understanding about your true feelings. It's common to write blindly and then reread your entries to find things about yourself that you didn't consciously realize before. In understanding your emotions, you can take the next step of coming to terms with them. It may be helpful to have a separate journal for each child that was aborted in your life, allowing you to identify the different emotions that may have accompanied each loss.

Again, writing letters you never intend to send is another way of expressing your feelings to people involved. Other activities that can help us cope include cooking, exercising, reading, playing a musical instrument, gardening, housecleaning, shopping, or just going to work.

When Others Don't Understand

You must remember that friends and family may find it difficult to understand the exact pain you are experiencing. Many husbands feel powerless to comfort their wives and suggest that they stop thinking about the abortion. Statements like "Don't bring up all that junk now—it will only cause you pain" are common in households where women are grieving. What they don't realize is that you aren't dredging up the pain—it's always with you like a knot in your throat. You can no longer deny its existence. In order to get through the pain, you must experience these emotions.

Try not to feel angry or rejected if your husband, family, or friends can't understand what you are going through. While these feelings can totally engross you, others calmly go on with life. They laugh and talk about trivial things while you writhe in agony. This can make you angry and frustrated. You want to run away from them and scream, but you discover that no matter where you go, your grief follows you. You may need to find a private place to open your heart without others interfering with this step of the healing process.

Individuals may expect you not to grieve, because it makes them uncomfortable. Maybe they have never had a loss, and they don't understand what you're feeling. In this circumstance you end up facing your grief alone. Try not to judge those who cannot help you.

After your season of grief is over, gently relay how you were feeling to them in an effort to educate them.

Other post-abortive women, if they haven't dealt with their own grief, can be the worst enemies of your mourning process. Keep in mind that if you share your grief with another PAS woman who is still in the denial stage of her emotions, she could easily discredit your feelings in order to fortify her own wall. She may also avoid you or try to dishonor you to others, fearful that you will reveal her secret. Unless you discover someone who is truly at your point in the grieving process, or further down the healing path, try not to confide in other post-abortive individuals.

Children have the hardest time understanding your feelings. Imagine if your mother started crying uncontrollably. Wouldn't you try to help her feel better any way you could? Your world revolves around this loved one and standing back while she is hurting is impossible. Remember that unless your children are adults, they simply cannot be burdened with this pain. Try to keep in control around young children. During a composed period, let them know that you are going through a hard time and that it has nothing to do with anything they have done. If restraint is impossible, ask a friend to baby-sit while you go out and have a good cry.

Give yourself the next few weeks or months to experience every emotion that comes your way. Try not to take on a new job or make a big move, but relax and accept the emotions as they come. Be assured that your feelings are normal and that you are physically unable to deny them any longer. Ask family and friends to be patient with you—this is your season of grief. Understand that it won't last forever, but that on the other side of the pain, there is peace.

Total grieving stops when we arrive in heaven, as outlined in Isaiah 60:20: "the LORD will be your everlasting light, and your days of sorrow will end." Isaiah 9:2 states, "The people walking in darkness have seen a great light; on those living in the land of the shadow of death a light has dawned." Revelation 7:17 says that God will "wipe away every tear from their eyes."

And in Psalm 56:8 (TLB), "You have seen me tossing and turning through the night. You have collected all my tears and preserved them in your bottle! You have recorded every one in your book."

Recognize that this period of grieving is precious to the Lord and helps rebuild your spiritual foundation with Him. He will take the responsibility for catching those tears and remembering them. God wants to use tears to release us from our pain.

I love you, O LORD, my strength.
The LORD is my rock, my fortress and my deliverer;
my God is my rock, in whom I take refuge.
He is my shield and the horn of my salvation, my
stronghold.
I call to the LORD, who is worthy of praise,
and I am saved from my enemies.
The cords of death entangled me;
the torrents of destruction overwhelmed me.
The cords of the grave coiled around me;
the snares of death confronted me.

In my distress I called to the LORD;
I cried to my God for help.
From his temple he heard my voice;
my cry came before him, into his ears.

—Psalm 18:1–6

Chapter 8

Joy Comes in the Mourning: Letting Go at Last

Forget the former things; do not dwell on the past.
See, I am doing a new thing! Now it springs up;
do you not perceive it?
I am making a way in the desert and streams
in the wasteland.
—Isaiah 43:18–19

Through the post-abortion-recovery class, I dealt with and found relief from the myriad emotions associated with my past. I felt as though I was shedding layer after layer of dead skin.

It was painful, but a new person was coming to life within me—a new person who was free! But there was one thing left to do. I had found the courage to face my emotions and release them; now it was time to face my long-lost baby ... and release him as well.

While it sometimes seems impossible to believe, there is a way to joy after an abortion. In mourning your loss, confessing your sin, forgiving yourself and others involved in your abortion decision, God's peace can come through and joy can once again fill your soul.

But there is one thing left to take care of; one more issue to confront. You've made things right with God; you've begun to forgive yourself; you're on the road to forgiving others … and now you need to make things right with your lost child. You need to answer the questions that plague your soul, and you need to say good-bye—at least, for now.

Confronting the Questions

It's one thing to deal with the tangible issues surrounding our abortions—feeling anger toward flesh-and-blood people; asking forgiveness from God whose Word assures us of His answer. But it's another thing altogether to come to the heart of what hurts … wondering what has happened to this child whom we were designed to protect, and how that baby regards us now. The questions are almost too frightening to face, but you'll never be fully at rest until you know the answers.

Where Is My Baby Now?

What a terrible guilt many struggle with because they are uncertain what happened to their babies! If a child dies before accepting Jesus, where does he go? Can she possibly find a home in heaven? How can we know for sure?

Scripture does address this issue. Jesus certainly welcomed

children. Remember when the disciples tried to keep the little ones from bothering Him? His response, in Matthew 19:14, was a rebuke: "Let the little children come to me, and do not hinder them, for the kingdom of heaven belongs to such as these."

This is a comforting passage to parents. But for the one who has aborted a child, an even more reassuring passage is found once again in 2 Samuel, the story of David and Bathsheba. If ever there was an unplanned pregnancy, theirs was. Soon after their child was born, the baby became gravely ill. David, finally aware of the tragedies he had set in motion, was wild with grief. He fasted and mourned for his son until, finally, the child died. Why did he stop then? Surely now his grief must be greater than ever. Second Samuel 12:22–23 tells us why. And his reason is one we, too, can cling to.

> While the child was still alive, I fasted and wept. I thought, "Who knows? The LORD may be gracious to me and let the child live." But now that he is dead, why should I fast? Can I bring him back again? I will go to him, but he will not return to me.

The hope in this verse is implied, but it is real nonetheless. David, certainly, expected to spend eternity in heaven, despite his sin. His many psalms tell of his absolute trust in God's mercy and forgiveness. As David states that he expects to go to his baby, he makes it clear that he believes his son is with the Lord in heaven. There was no debate—just calm assurance that he would see his boy again.

Solomon spoke about the unborn child that dies, in Ecclesiastes 6:3–6:

A man may have a hundred children and live many years;
yet no matter how long he lives, if he cannot enjoy his
prosperity and does not receive proper burial, I say that
a stillborn child is better off than he. It comes without
meaning, it departs in darkness, and in darkness its name
is shrouded. Though it never saw the sun or knew anything, it has more rest than does that man—even if he
lives a thousand years twice over but fails to enjoy his
prosperity. Do not all go to the same place?

Psalm 27:10 says, "Though my father and mother forsake me,
the LORD will receive me." And Matthew 18:10 states, "See that
you do not look down on one of these little ones. For I tell you
that their angels in heaven always see the face of my Father in
heaven."

God knows every heart that He's created. Like the old hymn
"Jesus Loves Me" says, "Little ones to Him belong. They are weak
but He is strong." Nowhere in Scripture is there a single verse
indicating that babies, even those conceived out of wedlock by
non-Christian parents, are unwelcome in the home of their heavenly Father. Rest assured that your little one is safe in the arms of
Jesus.

How Does My Baby Feel about Me?

Do you believe that your child might hate you for taking his or her
life? This is another common facet of the post-abortion experience.
There is often a deep dread of death, because it means we will come
face to face with the children we aborted. God is the only judge

in heaven—not our children—and you already know that He has offered His forgiveness to you.

In heaven there is no sorrow, judgment, or hatred—only joy filling each day, as outlined in Romans 14:17: "for the kingdom of God is not a matter of eating and drinking, but of righteousness, peace and joy in the Holy Spirit." Aborted children do not harbor bitterness against earthly inhabitants; they don't miss life on earth. Satan's grip is released in heaven and individuals are not plagued by the darkness that seeks to disrupt the Holy Spirit's peaceful presence in our hearts.

A human perspective on the aborted child's viewpoint comes from Christian recording artists Vince Lichlighter and Rob Yantis titled, "Please":

> Mommy, don't be crying, it's not hurting anymore
> I know the choice you must have made
> All of that is over now, but your pain remains
> And lots of things will never be the same
> I know you must have counted when my birthday
>   would've been
> I know at night you even hear me crying now and then
> I know you'd do it different, if it was all to do again
>
> Mommy, I'm beautiful, the angels here are too
> And you must know that I forgive you
> Mommy, Jesus told me that He loves you like I do
> And Jesus wants to meet you
> Mommy, Jesus told me that He loves you like I do
> And someday me and Jesus want to meet you.[1]

It's hard to know what heaven will be like exactly, but with God's help, you can know that your lost child will be very happy to meet you at last. Instead of dreading that day when you look in his eyes, you can look forward with joy to the moment you first hold her in your arms.

For many post-abortive women, it's very healing to sit down and write a letter to God that He can give to your child. By pouring out your sorrow directly to the child, apologizing, and acknowledging him or her as a human being, a vital step in mourning is accomplished. Had your child lived, he or she would have imparted great value upon the world and fulfilled a purpose God had designed just for that child. Realizing this at first deepens your grief, but in doing so, you can begin to mourn in the normal human fashion.

Mourning Your Loss

Mourning may not sound like a very pleasant proposition. It sounds like something that would deepen your grief, not lessen it! But the surprising thing is, mourning sets you free. Maybe that's why funerals and wakes and the like are such an intricate part of virtually every human culture—they help us accept and process the loss of something precious in our lives.

Around the time he would have been graduating from high school, I shed many more tears for my aborted child. Recently I have begun to grieve the grandchildren that my child might have been providing to my life. These emotions are normal and come with every loss. After Mac died, I'd find myself missing him in the most casual moments. These are

the same sentiments that I feel toward my child. I simply miss him, and, in those moments, tears come again.

Mourning and grief over the loss of your child will change over time as well. There are milestones that remind us of the period when our abortion occurred. When you aborted your baby, it's unlikely that you allowed yourself to consciously grieve. After all, who grieves the loss of a lump of tissue?

Give yourself the opportunity to mourn in a deliberate way. There is no prescribed formula for making this happen, however, so I'll walk through some suggestions later in this chapter. Whatever way you choose, you first will need to identify, at least to yourself, the person you are memorializing.

Giving Your Child a Name
When you have worked for years to keep the memory of the abortion away from your heart, thinking about the baby as a real human being is amazing. The simple task of giving your child a name is a great way to begin.

The post-abortion-recovery class suggested that we name our aborted children, but, though I was sure my baby was a boy, I couldn't name him, no matter how hard I tried. On the way to class I prayed, "Help me with this, Lord." Deep in my heart I heard His answer:

"Your son has been in heaven for eleven years. Don't you think I've named him by now? He's called Jesse."

That was it! His name was Jesse! It was simple and sweet. God had already named my son. He cares for every aborted child in heaven—enough to give them all a name when their parents couldn't even realize that they were children. And my son's name was special. It was King David's father's name—and Jesus was an adopted descendent from Jesse. God had cared enough to give my son a special name. I would later discover that Jesse means "God exists" in Hebrew.

Ways to Memorialize Your Child

Initially you may recoil from the thought of memorializing your child—it's probably not something you've imagined doing before. However, choosing a memorial as a way of remembering your child is an integral part of healing, although the tears may flow for days or weeks. There are as many different ways to memorialize a child as there are different children. You may want to hold a small, private funeral service; you might want to plant a tree; you may want to write a poem, make a donation to a charity in his name, write her story in a journal … the choice is purely personal.

When my mother's father passed away in 1968, she planted a very tiny magnolia tree in our backyard in his memory. Since her father's grave was in Ireland, she could not visit it during her grieving process. The tree was something she could look out on as she did the dishes each night and remember her father, and it was a comfort to her heart. Recently, a friend sent me a photo of this tree, which is now over forty years old. It has become tall and strong and was filled with incredible blossoms, the smell of which must have been amazing. While my grandfather has been dead for so long, the life of this special memorial is a gift to me and many others who never even knew him.

To memorialize their children, some women have purchased "mother's rings" with the birthstone of their aborted child. Others have purchased or created paintings that hang on the wall to remind them of this special person. Pressed flowers in a special book or journal are another, more private memorial. The memorial need not be obvious by any means. One woman planted three aspen trees in her backyard to represent her three children lost in abortion. The smallest items can provide comfort, and I hope you can find a memorial significant to you and your child.

When our post-abortion-recovery class leaders suggested that, as a group, we hold a memorial service for our aborted babies, most of us nearly fell off our chairs. I immediately vowed that I would not attend. Recognizing our lack of confidence, the leaders asked us to trust them that this would be a good experience. They suggested that we bring a candle for each baby and a bouquet of flowers.

The day of the service, I felt sick and stayed home from work to prepare. Michael's birth had been nine months earlier, and I had saved a wicker basket shaped like a bassinet from one of the flower arrangements I had received. From garden flowers, I made an arrangement with a candle-holder in the middle.

My husband wasn't sure that a memorial was such a good idea but offered to go along. Sensing his apprehension, I figured it would be better to go alone than to worry about his comfort during the service. Instead, I took my baby, Michael, with me. I felt that I needed a family member present. It's funny how much moral support young children can be!

*I carried Michael into the church and found the lighting and atmo-
sphere calming. I placed Jesse's bassinet basket on the altar and marveled
at how beautiful the arrangements looked. It was a peaceful place and I
was immediately at rest in my heart.*

*Music played quietly as the pastor began the service. Most cap-
tivating to me was his reading of John 11:43–44, about Lazarus:
"Jesus called in a loud voice, 'Lazarus, come out!' The dead man
came out, his hands and feet wrapped with strips of linen, and a
cloth around his face. Jesus said to them, 'Take off the grave clothes
and let him go.'"*

*The pastor then said, "I want to compare you to the risen Lazarus.
You are very much alive inside but still tightly bound by the grave
clothes—your children. We are simply here as friends to help you
remove these grave clothes."*

*As I sat there, I realized immediately that I had felt very bound
by Jesse's death. The pastor's analogy made perfect sense. I went to
pray with him, and he simply asked the Lord to remove these grave
clothes. Within that minute, I felt like I had lost thirty pounds! The
bondage of this sin was removed and I was free at last.*

*When I sat down, I hugged Michael closely and he quietly stayed
wrapped in my embrace for the remainder of the service. I had never
expected joy from this event—but that was what I was feeling. The
words to the old hymn became true in those following moments:*

> *Heaven came down and glory filled my soul*
> *When at the cross my Savior made me whole.*
> *My sins were washed away,*
> *And my night was turned to day.*
> *Heaven came down and glory filled my soul.[2]*

As I sat there, waiting for the other women to pray, I pondered what my child was feeling in heaven at that moment. For a brief second, as I closed my eyes, I saw what looked like the silhouette of a boy with his hands raised in the air as if he were cheering. I asked God what this was and felt an immediate response: "All of heaven is rejoicing; you've come home!" I couldn't help but wonder if the silhouette was my own Jesse cheering me on, saying, "Go, Mom!"

When you have experienced multiple abortions, healing may come harder. There are more memories, some deeply buried, and it simply takes longer to work them all through. You may want to follow the steps in this book separately for each abortion, since the situations and pain revolving around each experience can differ greatly. Likewise, you may want to memorialize each child separately, and perhaps differently as well.

Your Own Happy Ending

Certainly everyone is not able or required to have an actual funeral service for her children. Feel free to create something out of your own special talents. A tangible memorial can be very comforting—just like visiting the graveside of a beloved friend.

Whatever way you are led to remember your child, please step forward in faith and participate in some sort of memorial. As the years go by, it will remind you that you have honored your child, provided him or her with the human dignity of being named, and shed tears on the child's behalf. God's strong embrace through this process will strengthen and enrich your life and future relationships. And, most of all, it will bring you peace and hope for your future.

❋

A year later I felt led to put Jesse's name on a plaque at the National Memorial for the Unborn, in Chattanooga, Tennessee.[3] It was housed at a former abortion clinic, the very spot where thirty-five thousand children had passed into the arms of Jesus.

I marveled at the site of this special place and was reminded of Genesis 50:20: "You intended to harm me, but God intended it for good to accomplish what is now being done, the saving of many lives."

But I had only a first name for my son. I struggled with the knowledge that Jesse's father probably still did not mourn his loss and I felt using the father's last name wouldn't be appropriate.

Later my husband would finish Jesse's name in a quiet way. We were speaking about how I recognized his daughter from a previous marriage as my own. I reasoned that she was my son's sister, so that made her my child. No one could share the blood of my children and not be family. Tom simply said, "That's the way I think of Jesse. He's my son." Jesse finally had a full name. My mother paid the suggested donation for the plaque at the National Memorial for the Unborn and had only one request—that the word REDEEMED be on the third line.

....

I have set the LORD always before me.
Because he is at my right hand,
I will not be shaken.

Therefore my heart is glad and my tongue rejoices;
my body also will rest secure,
because you will not abandon me to the grave,
nor will you let your Holy One see decay.
You have made known to me the path of life;
you will fill me with joy in your presence,
with eternal pleasures at your right hand.

—Psalm 16:8–11

....

A good name is better than fine perfume,
and the day of death better than the day of
birth.
It is better to go to a house of mourning
than to go to a house of feasting,
for death is the destiny of every man;
the living should take this to heart.
Sorrow is better than laughter,
because a sad face is good for the heart.
The heart of the wise is in the house of mourning,
but the heart of fools is in the house of pleasure.

—Ecclesiastes 7:1–4

....

Chapter 9

Meeting in Paradise

Love has been perfected among us in this: that we
may have boldness in the day of judgment; because as
He is, so are we in this world. There is no fear in love;
but perfect love casts out fear, because fear involves
torment. But he who fears has not been made perfect
in love. We love Him because He first loved us.
—1 John 4:17–19 NKJV

There is one simple truth about abortion—our children are safe and warm in the arms of Jesus, the greatest parent a child could ever have. He calls them by name and they behold His beauty. This leads to the next obvious conclusion—if you want to meet your child someday, you must know Jesus Christ as your Savior. There is no true healing outside of the love of God and a relationship with Jesus Christ. Since your child is in heaven, you want to be there too!

God's Magnificent Obsession

When someone says, "God is love," we think, *What does that mean?*
Many people spend a great deal of time fearing God's wrath and judgment, but if 1 John 4:17–19, listed above, is truth, this fear of God is
wrong. There is no fear in love. I hadn't been "perfected" by God's love
until I could accept the love God gave me by sending His own Son to
earth to die for my sins. My recovery class leader said, "If your abortion was the only sin on earth, God still would have sent Jesus to die
on the cross." It's hard to comprehend love like that because we don't
understand the nature of God's love.

In 1 Corinthians 13, Paul talked about God's love as "agape"—
the kind that is based on the intentional decision of the one who
loves rather than the worthiness of the one who is loved. Part of our
misunderstanding of God's love is that we never felt worthy of it. But
God doesn't care how we feel—He loves us anyway.

God's form of love is written in 1 Corinthians 13. God's love is
faithful all the time and never proud or rude. God's love doesn't envy
and won't boast. God's love can't be angered and never thinks evil
thoughts about you. God's love doesn't rejoice in evil or injustice but
loves the truth. God's love bears, believes, endures, and hopes in all
things. God's love cannot fail you—ever.

When you lost your unborn child through abortion, His love
for you endured. As you fell into sin (promiscuity, drug abuse, and
so forth), He believed in you and knew that you were hurting. His
love waited for you.

He waited until you were able to bear the thought of your lost
child and turn to Him for help. His love watched over you during
your time in sin and protected you in spite of your choices. God

didn't care that you rejected Him. He wasn't leaving you, no matter what you did to push Him away. God's love doesn't care if you felt worthy, because He made you to be worthy. There has never been a moment in your existence that you could earn God's love, because He gave it to you when He conceived you in your mother's womb.

It's hard to understand that kind of love because there are so few examples on earth. That's because our world is full of humans. God isn't human and doesn't love that way. But He wants you to learn to love others in this same way. The most important part of healing is to understand God's love.

Perhaps you can't comprehend God's love right now. God loves you enough to help you understand this devotion. He will be patient, gentle, and kind with you. He will stand beside you as you cry or are angry with Him. There is nothing you can say or do that will turn Him away from loving you. You may as well just get used to the idea that He's going to teach you about His love in a way that few can comprehend.

Why are you so special? I don't know. I'm not God. He doesn't expect us to understand. What He wants is for me to talk to you about this love and plant the seed of hope in your heart that you have finally found the love you've been searching for. First Corinthians 13:13 (NKJV) says, "And now abide faith, hope, love, these three; but the greatest of these is love."

God loves you, no matter what. He truly does. Ask Him to help you know this love in your heart. If you don't feel anything, don't panic. He's there. It just may take Him a while to break down the walls of your heart to let His love shine in!

If God Loves Me, Why Doesn't He Just Take Away This Pain?

The answer to that question involves understanding that there were consequences for the decisions that you need to work through. He loved you enough to know that the process of grieving is good for your heart because it draws you closer to Him at a spiritual level. He can use it to teach you love for others going through the same pain.

We've all heard the proverb "Spare the rod and spoil the child." And we've all seen bratty kids. These are the ones whose parents don't discipline them. They run around creating havoc wherever they go, and people learn to dislike and avoid them. The lack of discipline means the child could face a tough future. Kids need boundaries and rules. In raising my own children, I have found how hard it is to discipline them when they are wrong. When I've told them, "This hurts me more than it hurts you," they've rarely believed me. But it's true. I hate to punish my kids. Yet in punishing them, I'm helping them understand authority and preparing them to live in society.

In Psalm 94:12–15 (NKJV) David wrote,

> Blessed is the man whom You instruct, O LORD,
> And teach out of Your law
> That You may give him rest from the days of adversity …
> For the LORD will not cast off His people,
> Nor will He forsake His inheritance.
> But judgment will return to righteousness,
> And all the upright in heart will follow it."

God's instruction for you now is to help you walk through the pain of your choices in life. He knows that if He just takes away your pain, you won't learn His love and healing. This pain is something that you will need to understand in order to avoid sin in the future.

In Hebrews 12:7–11 (NKJV) is another perspective:

> If you endure chastening, God deals with you as with sons; for what son is there whom a father does not chasten? But if you are without chastening, of which all have become partakers, then you are illegitimate and not sons. Furthermore, we have had human fathers who corrected us, and we paid them respect. Shall we not much more readily be in subjection to the Father of spirits and live? For they indeed for a few days chastened us as seemed best to them, but He for our profit, that we may be partakers of His holiness. Now no chastening seems to be joyful for the present, but painful; nevertheless, afterward it yields the peaceable fruit of righteousness to those who have been trained by it.

The only thing to do is to embrace this pain and understand that God is going to use it in your life, and that He doesn't enjoy watching you suffer. Many of you endured the wrong punishment from your parents. Pain can easily trigger horrible memories of the abuse of your past. If you experienced that type of pain, understand that chastisement was from a human and was wrong. God's discipline is holy and good. He will never give you more than you can handle. He knows your endurance because He created you.

Another thing to remember is that the pain is *temporary*. While you don't think it will ever go away, there are thousands of us on the other side of the pain to prove you wrong. We have survived the truth of our choices, grieved our losses, allowed God's love to help us forgive those who harmed us (including ourselves), and come to the point of peace where God can use us. Have hope that you won't feel this pain forever. Ask God to give you moments of peace to understand His love and discipline. He won't desert you—ever.

Praise the Lord in All Things

David glorified the Lord because God loved him in spite of his sin. In Psalm 8:3–5 (NKJV) he wrote,

> When I consider Your heavens, the work of Your fingers,
> The moon and the stars, which You have ordained,
> What is man that You are mindful of him,
> And the son of man that You visit him?
> For You have made him a little lower than the angels,
> And You have crowned him with glory and honor."

I remember thinking, *Who are you to think that you deserve to be loved by God?* As I looked into the smiling face of my second son, Michael, I marveled at the magnificence of God's creativity. Michael was just a few months old when I started the post-abortion recovery class. My heart always feared that because of my abortion God would punish me by taking the lives of my children. With my first son, Bruce, this fear prevented me from bonding with him completely—

if I kept my heart in check I wouldn't be hurt if something happened to him. This was wrong! God doesn't punish us like that. There may be physical consequences to our abortion, including infertility or miscarriages, but that isn't God's punishment.

There is no truth in any statement that begins with "God can't …" The incredible truth about grace is that God can do anything He wants to do. We can't put Him in a box or make ourselves worthy of His love. His love for us doesn't depend on our actions. He can love us even if we aren't repentant. He loves us even when we can't feel His love. We were handmade by Him! Every day of our lives was written in His book up in heaven. He knows our past, future, and present. He freely gives grace to all who come to Him humbly and acknowledge that "Jesus is Lord" and that He died on the cross for their sins. I'm really glad I don't have to carry my own sins on my shoulders, and I know I can never "earn" His love or a way to heaven. That is the amazing gift Jesus offers us—freedom from the burden of sin and guilt, and our inheritance as His sisters!

A friend of mine, Dr. Clarence Shuler, once said that he considered God his Daddy. While Clarence knew that he had made his father angry and had sinned, his status as his father's son never changed—only the relationship shifted. While many of us have earthly fathers who have abandoned us and may never embrace us again, God isn't like that at all! He's the true Father who loves and cares for *all* His children. Sometimes it's hard for us to understand because of our human nature and the bad examples of fatherhood before us.

One thing holding you back from God's love might be a fear that you will never feel as normal as you did before the abortion. Perhaps people have even told you that "complete" healing isn't possible. Isn't it nice to know that we don't have to rely on people's opinions when the Bible is the source of our truth? Love is not undone by sin, and abortion is not the "unpardonable sin." God sees all sin equally—no one is worse than another. And He loves us in spite of our sins—whether that's a lie or an abortion—because the price of our sin has already been paid for us in the sacrifice of Christ.

There is no one on earth who doesn't need Christ, and no one so bad that His sacrifice of love can't cover them. It's evident in Isaiah 53:2–5 (NKJV) where the prophet tells about the coming Christ:

> For He shall grow up before Him as a tender plant,
> And as a root out of dry ground.
> He has no form or comeliness;
> And when we see Him,
> There is no beauty that we should desire Him.
> He is despised and rejected by men,
> A Man of sorrows and acquainted with grief.
> And we hid, as it were, our faces from Him;
> He was despised, and we did not esteem Him.
> Surely He has borne our griefs
> And carried our sorrows;
> Yet we esteemed Him stricken,
> Smitten by God, and afflicted.
> But He was wounded for our transgressions,
> He was bruised for our iniquities;
> The chastisement for our peace was upon Him,
> And by His stripes we are healed.

God knows how you are feeling today. He knows those deep thoughts in your heart. He also knows the outcome of your life. You may feel like you are in pieces on the ground, but He knows how the pieces fit together. He marked out the grooves of how each circumstance in your life fits into who you are. He knows just how to assemble you.

Psalm 27:14 (NKJV) says, "Wait on the LORD; be of good courage, and He shall strengthen your heart. Wait, I say, on the LORD!" Are you waiting today? He's there, so take courage. Open your Bible and meet Him face-to-face in His Word; don't hide yourself from Him.

To find peace from your abortion experience, you need to have a relationship with Christ and the Father. His love is available to everyone—even (and maybe especially) His daughters who, like us, have chosen abortion. If you have never asked Jesus into your life, you can do so right now. The path of salvation is relayed in John 3:16 and Romans 10:9:

> For God so loved the world that he gave his one and only Son, that whoever believes in him shall not perish but have eternal life.

> That if you confess with your mouth, "Jesus is Lord," and believe in your heart that God raised him from the dead, you will be saved.

Do you want an intimate relationship with Jesus? These scriptures are your blueprint for salvation. Open your heart and believe in Him.

God's Unlimited Patience

If you accepted Christ as your Savior after your abortion decision, you may understand the powerful cleansing of this sin that occurred in your salvation experience. While there still may be issues that need to be addressed, the Lord's grace and mercy has the power to set us free instantly.

If you, like me, made the abortion decision as a Christian, don't believe Satan's accusing lie that your sin is greater as a result. The accuser's voice can also be magnified when you made more than one abortion decision. As a child, I had a plaque in my room that read, "Please be patient. God isn't finished with me yet." We are all human beings on common ground and fully capable of sinful actions. We can draw comfort from the fact that when we met the Lord, He forgave our past, present, and future sins.

I know that the Holy Spirit attempted to get my attention with the truth of His special gift of my unplanned pregnancy. Ignoring His voice had different consequences, and the wall within my heart was stronger, compounded by the fact that I should have known better. Even in that understanding, God was merciful. He knew my heart didn't understand the decision I was making or the consequences for the rest of my life.

After my abortion, I silenced the beautiful voice of the Holy Spirit; when I left that clinic, I could not bear to approach the Lord in prayer again. Instead I listened to the voice of Satan, who assured me that God would never want me again now that I'd taken the life of His created child.

Nearly four years after the abortion, with extensive promiscuity and drug dependency still existing in my life, I began to truly miss God. I longed for the comfort of the Holy Spirit. But I didn't know how to find my way back to Him. I was so overwhelmed with the sins before me and ashamed. What if He didn't want me back?

I had just graduated from college and moved to California to start a new life with a friend from college, Susan. My heart wanted to put aside the party and begin to address my career. Unfortunately I found myself in a worse environment in California, with more drugs and a deeper level of decadence.

After six long days in that uncomfortable environment, I went outside and looked at the stars. I needed and wanted God. I said a very quick prayer: "God, if You have a husband out there for me, he could show up any time." Unbeknownst to me, with that small prayer I asked for God's help, and the bricks at the foundation of the wall in my heart were blasted out. God heard my prayer and His love began to seep into my wounded heart.

As many of us do, I took one step forward and four steps back. After the abrupt prayer, Susan's roommate came outside and said, "You look sad. Let's go out and get drunk." Not knowing what else to do, I agreed. The next morning I found myself in bed with a man who had the reputation of "bedding" every new girl who came to town. I was overwhelmed and shocked at myself because I had never sunk that low before. Sadly, I recollected little of the evening before and nothing about what went on with the virtual stranger lying next to me.

I fled back to Susan's apartment. How could I have prayed and then done such a horrible thing? But still I felt the hand of God on my heart at a much stronger level.

*That evening found me in deeper depression and remorse. Not know-
ing what else to do, I went to the restaurant where Susan was tending
bar. The cook from the restaurant sat down next to me. I had met him
earlier that week, but his smiling face was no comfort. Then he said, "I
heard you were with Monterrey Ray last night." Tears immediately came
to my eyes.*

*Seeing my pain at his comment, this man was immediately apolo-
getic. He spent the next ten minutes expressing remorse to make up for
his insensitivity. He worked so hard to make me feel better that he got
my attention. I allowed myself a moment to look into his eyes and saw a
different level of compassion there than I had ever seen before.*

*I suddenly heard the Lord's voice in my heart, saying, "You asked Me
about your husband last night, didn't you? Well, here he is...." My heart
stumbled for a moment with the beauty of understanding that in spite
of all my choices and sins, God had not only heard my prayer but had
answered it as well. These compassionate eyes belonged to my husband,
Tom. I asked him about God and he smiled broadly, saying, "I know
the Lord. I'm a Christian...." A few weeks later, when I told him about
my abortion, I would fall in love with him five hundred percent more
because he offered me godly love and acceptance. My healing didn't come
overnight, but from then on, Tom was by my side, patiently showing me
the Lord.*

Sometimes all it takes is a small and simple "Help me, God" prayer to
discover the Lord's voice in your heart. While God has never left your
side, your wall of protection may have held Him waiting outside of
your heart's door. God is a gentleman. He won't come in unless He's
invited! Are you ready to invite Him to come in? Luke 11:9–10 relays

this truth: "Ask and it will be given to you; seek and you will find; knock and the door will be opened to you. For everyone who asks receives; he who seeks finds; and to him who knocks, the door will be opened." "Help me, God...." is the prayer to humbly make in your heart right now. Then be ready to record the ways He begins to restore your soul, answering each and every prayer in His good time.

If you were a Christian at the time of your abortion like I was, find hope in 1 Timothy 1:12–17, "I thank Christ Jesus our Lord, who has given me strength, that he considered me faithful, appointing me to his service. Even though I was once a blasphemer and a persecutor and a violent man, I was shown mercy because I acted in ignorance and unbelief. The grace of our Lord was poured out on me abundantly, along with the faith and love that are in Christ Jesus."

Here is a trustworthy saying that deserves full acceptance: Christ Jesus came into the world to save sinners—of whom I am the worst. But for that very reason I was shown mercy so that in me, the worst of sinners, Christ Jesus might display his unlimited patience as an example for those who would believe on him and receive eternal life. Now to the King eternal, immortal, invisible, the only God, be honor and glory for ever and ever. Amen.

....

Out of the depths I cry to you, O LORD;
O Lord, hear my voice.
Let your ears be attentive
to my cry for mercy.

If you, O LORD, kept a record of sins,
  O Lord, who could stand?

But with you there is forgiveness;
  therefore you are feared.

I wait for the LORD, my soul waits,
  and in his word I put my hope.

My soul waits for the Lord
more than watchmen wait for the morning,
more than watchmen wait for the morning.

O Israel, put your hope in the LORD,
  for with the LORD is unfailing love
  and with him is full redemption.

He himself will redeem Israel
  from all their sins.

—Psalm 130:1–8

Chapter 10

Where Do I Go from Here?

He has sent me to bind up the brokenhearted, to
proclaim freedom for the captives and release from
darkness for the prisoners … to comfort all who
mourn, and provide for those who grieve in Zion—
to bestow on them a crown of beauty instead of
ashes, the oil of gladness instead of mourning, and
a garment of praise instead of a spirit of despair.
—Isaiah 61:1–3

A few years after my healing, a call came through the counseling
lines at Focus on the Family, and the phone was handed to me. It was
a woman who was considering abortion. What on earth was I to say to
her? Terror filled my heart as I realized my words might be the only thing

standing between this child and death. I said a quick prayer and listened as she told me her story.

She was pregnant from a one-night encounter, and she was already the single mother of three girls. One of her daughters was thirteen, and the mother was afraid that if her daughter found out about the pregnancy, all hope of her choosing an abstinent lifestyle would be gone.

I shared with this woman about the pain that abortion brings and prayed with her, but as we hung up, she still leaned toward ending the pregnancy. For two weeks, another post-abortive woman and I prayed for this mother and called her frequently. The day before her abortion appointment, she was still planning to go through with it. We prayed fervently for her that evening, and the next day, when we called, she was at home! She had changed her mind at the last minute.

Seven months later, a message on my desk contained these words about this woman's delivery:

It's a boy!

7 lbs. 9 oz.

19 inches long

His name is Jesse!

This mother had no idea what I had named my lost son, but her little Jesse was proof positive that my Jesse had not died in vain.

If reading through these chapters has touched your heart, then many prayers have been answered. In the warmth and security of your own home, God has come down into your heart and begun the work of His healing. But your journey doesn't end here.

Continuing Your Own Healing

You have done a lot of work in your heart since you began reading this book. You have likely shed many tears, fought through much pain, and dredged up many memories you'd tried to forget. An experience like abortion is not an easy one to put behind you.

You've made a wonderful start on the road to healing, and a brave one. Probably you are feeling a greater degree of peace than you have sensed in a long time. But there is no comfort like that which you can receive from God's people—the brothers and sisters in Christ who have also survived an abortion experience. I encourage you to join a post-abortion recovery class and experience the bond that shared grief can bring. The women there will understand a part of you that has lived in isolation since the day of your abortion.

Currently there are more than two thousand pregnancy care centers in the United States. They provide free pregnancy tests, limited medical services, abstinence education, maternity and baby clothes, furniture, housing, parenting classes, and friendship. Another tier of their service is in the area of reconciliation—post-abortion ministry. Most are located under the "Abortion Alternatives" section of the yellow pages or on the "Find Help" section of RamahInternational.org. Call and ask them about their post-abortion ministry. In most cases, your call will be completely confidential and you will be treated with love, compassion, and care.

After you visit the center, pray about joining whatever program they offer on post-abortion trauma. Ask specifically to be introduced to other post-abortive individuals and strike up friendships wherever possible. Also, begin to put out some feelers within your own circle of friends. The Alan Guttmacher Institute (Planned Parenthood's

former research group) estimated that 33 percent of American women
have had at least one abortion by the age of forty-five.[1] Chances are
good that you know some of them! The blessings that will come from
these relationships will be treasures to you in the years to come. And
as you continue to work through your abortion issues, remember
Philippians 1:6: "He who began a good work in you will carry it on
to completion."

Participating in Others' Healing

Imagine yourself, back at the time of your unplanned pregnancy,
walking into a Christian center that provided you with an accurate
picture of the consequences of abortion. Should you have been fearful of your parents' reaction, the compassionate women there would
have gone with you to help you break the news. At all points in
your pregnancy, they would have stood by you and offered help and
friendship. These gracious, God-fearing individuals would also have
been there as you delivered your precious baby into the world. They
would have helped you get started raising your little one, or would
have supported you during an adoption process.

Wouldn't that have been better than the alternative you ended
up with? You can be that compassionate, gracious, God-fearing person for another woman.

Many of you have cried multitudes of tears since first opening the
cover of this book. Though there may be more healing yet to come
in your life, already you have something to offer other women, who,
like yourself, have experienced the pain and regret of abortion. And
you certainly have much to offer women who are at the crossroads,
facing an unplanned pregnancy and uncertain what to do.

Can you imagine the incredible feeling of holding a baby that God used you to save? To know that this baby would have surely died and God intervened with your testimony to save her life is a joy few realize in a lifetime. Whatever your gifts, whether you are good at public speaking, raising money, teaching classes, organizing workers, folding baby blankets, or drying tears, God can use you. And pregnancy care centers across the country have a place for you.

Ramah International offers seminars and conferences across the world in the area of post-abortion ministry development. Pregnancy care centers have an extensive training program for their volunteer counseling staff. Most also offer prayer coverage and friendship to every volunteer regardless of their role. The Lord's presence is very powerful in these centers and His ministry through you can be one of the most rewarding in your life.

You may be surprised how God provides opportunities to participate in the healing of other women. However He does it, God can use you for His ultimate purpose of healing.

Future Healing

There was a great deal more healing to be accomplished in my heart after the recovery class was completed. Initially, I felt lost without the constant support of the group. I was hoping that many would remain friends, but life happens, and we all were ready to put our abortions behind us. The pregnancy center invited me to lead the next group and I gratefully accepted the offer.

In that group we had a young woman who was very pregnant. She wasn't married and had an abortion in her past. I loved her immediately, but the staff wasn't sure how the other group members would respond to her pregnancy. For many post-abortive individuals, pregnant women are a reminder of their own loss. I pushed them to consider her because I knew she wouldn't have time to attend the class after her baby's birth. Without the healing the class could provide, her bonding skills with this new infant could be impacted—helping her heal seemed urgent. The class members adopted her, gave her a baby shower, and showed up at the hospital to see her child. It helped their healing and mine to love her and meet her baby.

One particular woman came to two classes and, after she shared her testimony, determined never to return. Her psychologist had forced her to come, and she really didn't want to do the work. It wasn't her time to address this pain because she still felt abortion had been her best decision. Another woman was struggling with sexual abuse. Still another had aborted because the baby was a child of rape. One woman didn't cry a tear until the memorial service. She'd had her abortion when she was thirteen, at her parents' insistence. At the memorial service, her parents cried with her.

While there are so many "faces" to post-abortion trauma, the eventual pain afterward can be much the same. Over the years, I have been granted great discernment on the post-abortive perspective. After speaking with thousands, I've learned how similar our pain really is. Many want to help others but perhaps it isn't their season of helping. Others just don't feel like God wants them in the field. Some are directed to other areas of ministry. The big part of this is determining what God wants you to do through prayer and reading His Word. My role today is much different than it was in 1991. God seems to shift and change us as the years pass by. One thing is for sure—He never wastes our pain or our experience. They are always part of the next phase of work.

God's Advance Work

Two years prior to my leaving Focus on the Family to start Ramah International, God gave me the vision for this current ministry. There have been many days that I have lamented not stepping out in faith sooner, but I realize that God built His plan in my heart and gave me time to get used to it. He had a specific timetable in place and knew my human mind had to prepare.

God woke me up in the night with a simple statement to my heart that said, "Help the post-abortive." It was such a vivid message and I immediately started thinking, "I'm doing that now at Focus on the Family in many ways." I didn't hear any response, but I had a strong feeling that this message meant for me to help the post-abortive on a full-time basis instead of just haphazardly. Yet it didn't sound like a good proposition financially, so I put it out of my mind and tried to fall back to sleep.

Over the following months God would bring people into my path to confirm the need for a person in full-time post-abortion international ministry. Then came a call from the leader of one of the main post-abortion referral agencies. She questioned me on my belief that the final destination of aborted babies was heaven, disagreeing that we should offer this hope to women. I calmly asked, "Well, if babies aren't in heaven, where are they?" She responded quickly, "I'm not sure, but wouldn't it be a great deterrent to abortion if women thought their babies were going to hell?" Her words drove cold shivers down my spine. She wasn't describing the Creator that I knew in my heart. In fact, her philosophy could certainly damage post-abortive individuals and leave them in deeper bondage to guilt and shame.

God continued to wake me up at night on a consistent basis to push my mind to embrace His calling. I believe Ramah began in a simple desire for me to sleep through the night! He gave me the name of the ministry and its biblical basis on the way home from work (see pages 183–188) and I finally gave in.

While many people—including extended family members—didn't understand the call to leave my well-respected national position at Focus on the Family to venture into the shaky world of nonprofit development, God was adamant. He wanted our trust and faith in His leading. Years later I look back and consider my human heart and am thankful that God pushed me to do His will in spite of my reluctance. It's been an incredible time of reaching wounded hearts, working with women, and helping develop much-needed resources. He has been our provider and leader each and every day. Psalm 138:8 (NKJV) says, "The LORD will perfect that which concerns me; Your mercy, O LORD, endures forever."

Taming Triggers

Second Corinthians 10:4–5 outlines the spiritual warfare and victory we may encounter as a result of this choice in the future,

> The weapons we fight with are not the weapons of the world. On the contrary, they have divine power to demolish strongholds. We demolish arguments and every

pretension that sets itself up against the knowledge of God, and we take captive every thought to make it obedient to Christ.

Approaching anniversary dates led me to refresh my heart with the knowledge of God's forgiveness through in-depth Scripture reading. I have learned to expect and embrace "mourning moments" around the time my child would have been born. I've discovered these same emotions when milestones would have been reached in his life: graduating from high school and college, giving me grandchildren, and so on. Even after all these years, I try to make that week as positive as possible, understanding that the grief may come again.

When I go to the dentist's office, I'm careful to take along music and a headset to drown out the sound of the drill, which can transport me back to the abortion experience. Should music come on the radio from that period, or when a particular aroma that reminds me of those days, I'm careful to "take every thought captive" and no longer be bound to shame, anxiety, and guilt. God has helped me to understand triggers of pain and to become victorious in the peace that He continues to provide my heart.

If the old emotions of regret and shame return to your heart, remember that you are not the same person you were when you made the abortion decision—consciously remember that fact. Take these thoughts captive as well, reminding yourself that you have become a new creature in the Lord. He has made you His bride, restoring the virgin status to your heart and covering you with His love. This is outlined in Revelation 21:4–7 (NKJV):

"God will wipe away every tear from their eyes; there shall be no more death, nor sorrow, nor crying. There shall be no more pain, for the former things have passed away." Then He who sat on the throne said, "Behold, I make all things new.... I will give of the fountain of the water of life freely to him who thirsts. He who overcomes shall inherit all things, and I will be his God and he shall be My son."

Rest in the peace of being a new creature in Christ.

Ways to Help

There are many things you can do when the Lord has healed your heart. Here are some tangible ways you can be involved in positive-life efforts:

Give

- Give this book and other positive life topic resources to your public, church, and school libraries.
- Donate baby items to pregnancy care centers.
- Offer gently used maternity clothes to pregnancy care centers.
- Contribute money to pregnancy care centers in honor of or in memory of friends.
- Financially support a pregnancy care center.

Educate

- Teach your children to say no to sex in a practical and understandable manner.

- Be informed on life issues: abortion, infanticide, euthanasia, stem-cell research, fetal experiments, etc.
- As the Lord leads, discuss the abortion issue with friends, always offering compassion and hope in the expectation that your audience may be post-abortive.
- Help your children write and talk at school about positive-life issues (science, current events, English paper, etc.).

Do

- Use your creative talents to create baby and other items for pregnancy care centers.
- Make a gift bag of small baby items for a new mother.
- Use positive-life resource cards and stationary.
- Wear "precious feet" pins that outline the size of a baby's feet at ten weeks' gestation.
- Call in to talk shows that are discussing life issues, and express your opinion, offering the hope of God's healing to wounded listeners.
- Patronize companies that support your local pregnancy care center.
- If there isn't a pregnancy care center in your area, organize a committee of positive-life-minded individuals to consider the possibility of starting one.
- Use physicians who don't refer or perform abortions.
- Offer your special talents to assist the work of pregnancy centers.
- Volunteer to do general office work at a pregnancy care center.

- Take meals and offer babysitting services to a single mom or caregiver.
- Vote for positive-life-minded candidates at all levels of the judicial system.

Write

- Write letters to newspapers expressing your positive-life perspective on abortion and carefully outline the hope for healing after this choice.
- Write letters to legislators expressing your personal perspective on abortion with suggestions on ways they can help individuals who are wounded by this choice.
- Write letters of encouragement to pregnancy care leaders.
- Write notes of cheer to the elderly, sick, or newly single parents.
- Circulate and sign petitions designed to promote legislation to reduce the number of abortions (i.e., informed consent legislation, embryonic stem-cell issues).

Pray

- Pray daily for your local pregnancy care center.
- Pray for expecting single mothers.
- Pray for those who are employed in the abortion industry.
- Pray for legislators.

Requiring More Commitment
- Always thank God for your children.

- Receive training to enable you to open your home to a pregnant mother.
- Become a foster parent.
- Offer to baby-sit for a disabled child.
- Share about your abortion experience to close friends.
- Run for political office to enhance the positive-life perspective in all areas of society.
- Become a board member for a pregnancy care center.
- Donate childcare to single parents.
- Provide a night out, a weekend or week vacation to a caregiver of the elderly, sick, or disabled.
- Involve a single mother or caregiver in your family activities and holiday events.

If you aren't sure of what God wants you to do, don't worry about it—just continue to pray for His direction. He'll be very obvious in His time. Whatever the Lord leads you to do, I encourage you to continue to seek Him daily in His Word and through prayer. Connect to a body of positive-life believers that can support you and provide insight and encouragement. Contact your local pregnancy care center and sign up for their post-abortion recovery program.

Keep in mind the words of David in Psalm 41:11–13 (NKJV),

By this I know that You are well pleased with me,
Because my enemy does not triumph over me.
As for me, You uphold me in my integrity,
And set me before Your face forever.

Blessed be the LORD God of Israel
From everlasting to everlasting!
Amen and Amen."

....

Be at rest once more, O my soul,
for the LORD has been good to you....
How can I repay the LORD
for all his goodness to me?
I will lift up the cup of salvation
and call on the name of the LORD.
I will fulfill my vows to the LORD
in the presence of all his people.
Precious in the sight of the LORD
is the death of his saints.
O LORD truly I am your servant;...
you have freed me from my chains.
I will sacrifice a thank offering to you
and call on the name of the LORD.

—Psalm 116:7, 12–17

....

Afterword

Stephen Arterburn

You may find it strange that this book would end with words from a man. I hope you will not allow my gender to prevent you from reading further. You may have some very strong feelings about men because of past treatment or perhaps how your father raised you. Many men do not have a good record when it comes to our treatment of others.

I am writing to you because I pressured someone much like you into having an abortion. I made sure she knew I would not be there for her and the baby if she chose to have it. I never gave her one ounce of hope that I could be swayed to commit to her or the child that I had helped to create.

I became an iron wall of resistance to any thought of becoming a responsible man, husband, or father. Even the idea of her having the baby and placing it up for adoption was an insult to the plans I had contrived for myself. That wonderful young lady and that baby growing in her womb were of little significance to me compared to the grand plans I had for myself. I wanted this inconvenience out of the way and did everything I could to ensure that the abortion took place. It did, and although I have received Christ's forgiveness that has freed me from this horrible choice, to this day I live with a painful regret that my child never was and never will be here on earth.

When I have spoken about the abortion to other men, they have often told me about their experiences. Some have wept openly. They too have feelings of doubt, regret, and shame, and have paid a stiff penalty for a choice that is so easily made in haste. Like me, they now look forward to a day in heaven when they can be with the child that was meant to be, but never was. The fellowship of their suffering is little comfort to me. It is only confirmation that many men like me owe women like you a great debt of apology and need to make restitution.

I write these words as a small offering to you from all men who shirked their duty and lived the life of common irresponsibility. Please forgive us where we have failed you.

God will restore you and renew your strength. You can trust God with your pain, your fears, and your future. When you experience His grace, you will be surprised by God. You will be amazed at His strength and astounded by His gentleness.

My hope for you is that *Her Choice to Heal* has been a book of truth and healing. I pray that you have found a new life and future in the arms of a God of not just second chances, but One of third, fourth, fifth chances and beyond. I pray that you will move through the pain and suffering and into what God can do through you. Take the comfort you have been given and commit your life to dispensing comfort to those who find themselves locked in similar situations.

May you receive the truth with grace from the God who has loved even the thought of you for millions of years.

A Final Note:
The Ministry of Ramah International

Founded in 1997 by Sydna A. Massé, Ramah International is based on Jeremiah 31:15–17. The need for Ramah International is based on 15:

> A voice is heard in Ramah, mourning and great weeping, Rachel weeping for her children and refusing to be comforted, because her children are no more.

The research arm of Planned Parenthood (the world's largest abortion provider), the Alan Guttmacher Institute, states that at least half of American women will experience an unintended pregnancy by age forty-five, and, at current rates, about one-third will have had an abortion.[1] Clearly, the post-abortive represent a large segment of our society. Yet few confess to this sin, especially to family and friends. Many deny comfort because they fear rejection and/or are unable to confront their own participation in ending their child's life. Except for a handful of small ministry efforts offered through our nation's two thousand pregnancy care centers and direct ministries, little is being done to reach these hearts with forgiveness and healing comfort available through Jesus Christ.

The solution that Ramah International can provide our world is based on Jeremiah 31:16:

This is what the LORD says, "Restrain your voice from
weeping and your eyes from tears, for your work will be
rewarded. [Your children] will return from the land of
the enemy."

Ramah International's purpose is to bring individuals struggling
with post-abortion syndrome to God's healing so they can cease
mourning by finally grieving their children's deaths and live normal
lives. It is heartbreaking work to touch this pain, yet helping them to
acknowledge the loss of their children is the first step to post-abortion
syndrome healing, and their "work will be rewarded." When a person
suffering from post-abortion syndrome names her child, the child
becomes a permanent part of his or her parents' heart. In essence,
they are redeemed from Satan's grasp and "return from the land of
the enemy."

The result of Ramah International's work is based on Jeremiah
31:17:

"So there is hope for your future," declares the LORD.

What is the hope for someone suffering from post-abortion
syndrome? For many, it is to stop abortion from hurting other lives.
Post-abortive individuals are strong voices who can attest to the
fact that abortion is a horrible choice—not only for the mother but
also for the child. They are excellent in ministering to the abortion-
minded individual.

Ministry Objectives

While the need for post-abortion syndrome (PAS) resources is substantial, currently there are very few resources available to assist those living with PAS. While pregnancy care centers (PCCs) have been active in this ministry, few churches have developed effective ministries to help the post-abortive. Ramah's plan is to work with the available PCC and PAS ministries to develop and provide resources necessary to restore the lives of these people and to minister to the abortion-minded.

We believe significant benefits will be realized as Ramah achieves its goals:

- Lives will be restored. Personal and family relationships will be restored. Personal relationships with God will be restored.
- As these lives are restored, these people will be able to reach others—especially the abortion-minded.
- Once restored, a substantial percentage of these people will become advocates within the positive-life community. It is the voices of the healed post-abortive individuals that will eventually awaken our world to the destruction of abortion.

Ramah International, Inc. is a nonprofit positive-life ministry whose mission is as follows:

- reach the post-abortive with the hope of God's healing;
- educate the abortion-minded with the truth of abortion's devastation;

- raise the level of awareness about the needs of individuals who have experienced abortion;
- provide post-abortion resources, research, and training programs necessary to mobilize and equip the church to reach out and help those affected by abortion so that post-abortive individuals can become involved in helping others who are considering or have experienced abortion;
- encourage the work of pregnancy care centers as they minister to the wounded.

Ramah's work includes
- resource development, including recovery guides, books, training manuals, devotionals, tracts, videos, newsletters, etc.;
- training programs to equip pregnancy care centers, church leaders, and counselors in post-abortion and abortion-minded ministry;
- media campaigns that educate on the pain after abortion and offer compassionate support and referrals to those wounded by this choice;
- an interactive Web site (RamahInternational.org) that offers information, resources, and referrals for those considering abortion, struggling after the choice, ministering to individuals, and impacted by an abortion decision;
- establishment and support of international pregnancy center and post-abortion efforts involving translated resources, training, and Web sites.

Ramah International's vision is to

- build awareness of post-abortion syndrome in the culture to a point where the majority is aware of its impact;
- reach people affected by post-abortion syndrome (i.e., mothers, fathers, grandparents, siblings, individuals who participated in abortion decision), offering them the hope of God's healing;
- educate the abortion-minded individual as to the spiritual, physical, psychological, and emotional aspects of abortion and provide them with referrals to local pregnancy care centers;
- train post-abortive individuals, pregnancy care center leaders, church leaders, Christian counselors, missionaries, etc. to reach the hearts of the abortion-minded and post-abortive individuals with God's healing;
- provide resources that will assist trained leaders in ministering to post-abortive and abortion-minded individuals (i.e., recovery guides, tracts, videos, newsletters, etc.);
- provide communication channels (i.e., Internet Web site, etc.) that provide abortion-minded and post-abortive individuals with a safe, confidential medium to reach out for help;
- offer a Web site for pregnancy care centers and individuals to encourage, education, inform, and network their efforts;
- through research, provide tangible evidence that post-abortion syndrome exists among those who have chosen the abortion option.

Please visit our Web site at RamahInternational.org to learn more about our current ministry training schedule and resources. The opportunity for you to be involved in helping share the joy of healing with other post-abortive individuals is available, and we pray you will consider joining our efforts.

All donations to Ramah International are tax-deductible and gratefully appreciated. Your gift will allow us to extend God's hope and healing to other hurting individuals. We would love to hear how this recovery guide has affected your healing. Please feel free to e-mail, write, or call at the following address:

Sydna A. Massé
Ramah International
1776 Hudson St.
Englewood, FL 34223
941-473-2188
941-473-2248 (fax)
e-mail: Sydna@aol.com—RamahInternational.org

May God continue to bless you and minister to your needs!

Notes

PROLOGUE

1. Facts on Induced Abortion in the United States, The Alan Guttmacher Institute, January, 2008, www.guttmacher.org/pubs/fb_induced_abortion. html#5.
2. Anne C. Speckhard and Vincent M. Rue, "Post-Abortion Syndrome: An Emerging Public Health Concern," *Journal of Social Issues*, 48, no. 3 (1992).

CHAPTER 1: My Abortion Story

1. Facts on Induced Abortion in the United States, The Alan Guttmacher Institute, January, 2008, www.guttmacher.org/pubs/fb_induced_abortion. html#5.

CHAPTER 2: What Is Post-Abortion Syndrome?

1. Frederica Mathewes-Green, *Policy Review*, Summer (1991).
2. Speckhard and Rue, "Post-Abortion Syndrome."
3. C. Everett Koop: Letter to President Ronald Reagan concerning the health effects of abortion. Medical and Psychological Impact of Abortion. Washington: U.S. Government Printing Office, 1989; 9: 68–71.
4. "Report of the American Psychological Association Task Force on Mental Health and Abortion," August 13, 2008, http://www.apa.org/releases/ abortion-report.pdf (accessed August 14, 2008).
5. http://www.thenation.com/directory/bios/sarah_blustain.
6. http://www.thenation.com/doc/20080204/blustain (accessed August 14, 2008).
7. http://www.utne.com/2008-04-04/Politics/Parsing-Post-Abortion-Syndrome-in-Men.aspx?blogid=30 (accessed August 14, 2008).
8. www.prochoiceamerica.org/assets/files/Abortion-Access-to-Abortion-Science-Post-Ab_Syndrome.pdf, January 1, 2008.
9. Paul and Teri Reisser, *Help for the Post Abortive Woman* (Lewiston, NY: Life Cycle Books, 1989), 35.
10. Speckhard and Rue, "Post-Abortion Syndrome."

CHAPTER 3: A Wall of Denial

1. C. S. Lewis, *The Four Loves* (New York: Harcourt Brace Jovanovich, Inc., 1960), 169.
2. quote from www.timesonline.co.uk/tol/life_and_style/health/article3559486. ece

3. Warren W. Wiersbe, *The Wiersbe Bible Commentary: Old Testament*, (Colorado Springs: David C. Cook, 2007), 913.
4. *American Heritage Dictionary*, New College Edition, v.v. "shame."
5. Speckhard and Rue, "Post-Abortion Syndrome."

CHAPTER 4: Bitter Roots: Anger
1. H. Norman Wright, *Crisis Counseling* (San Bernardino, CA: Here's Life Publishers, 1985), 285.
2. Ibid.
3. Speckhard and Rue, "Post-Abortion Syndrome."
4. Chapter 5, "The Heart of the Matter: Forgiveness," also deals with anger.

CHAPTER 5: The Heart of the Matter: Forgiveness
1. American Heritage Dictionary, s.v. "forgive."
2. C. S. Lewis, *Letters to Malcolm: Chiefly on Prayer* (New York: Harcourt Brace Jovanovich, Inc., 1964), 27.

CHAPTER 6: Sharing the Secret of Abortion
1. "Asleep in the Light," words and music by Keith Green, 1978 Birdwing Music/Cherry Lane Music Publishing Co., Inc./Ears to Hear Music. (www.KeithGreen.com)

CHAPTER 8: Joy Comes in the Mourning: Letting Go at Last
1. "Please," by Vince Lichlighter and Rob Yantis. Used by permission.
2. John W. Peterson, "Heaven Came Down" (John W. Peterson Music Co.: 1961, 1989). Used by permission.
3. www.memorialfortheunborn.org.

CHAPTER 10: Where Do I Go from Here?
1. An Overview of Abortion in the United States (The Alan Guttmacher Institute: January 2008).

A FINAL NOTE
1. "Facts on Induced Abortion in the United States," The Alan Guttmacher Institute, January 2008, www.guttmacher.org/pubs/fb_induced_abortion.html#5.